THE TWO PILLARS OF POWER

REIN IN YOUR PHYSICAL HEALTH AND MENTAL HEALTH TO SUPERCHARGE YOUR LIFE IN LESS THAN 7 DAYS

B&V HEALTHY LIVING

ABOUT THE AUTHOR

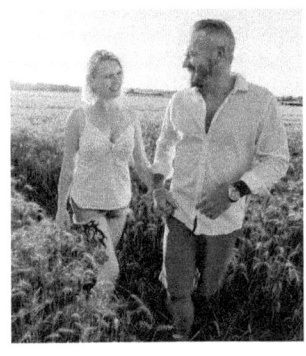 Brian and Vanda of B&V Healthy Living are passionate about helping people improve their quality of life. They endorse an organic lifestyle centered around European practices like growing your own fruit and vegetables, walking and biking, connecting with nature, and eating a healthy and balanced diet. Vanda promotes a healthy and happy mindset of daily affirmations, self-care and self-love, healthy eating, banishing negativity and focusing on positivity, and improving mental health. Throughout their marriage, they have experienced life's ups and downs, the many changes and challenges that the modern world presents, and have combined their knowledge and growth to create a motivational and inspirational company that helps people to live with positivity, purpose, and good health. Check out their blog and find out more about them at **www.bvhealthyliving.com**.

CONTENTS

JUST FOR YOU!

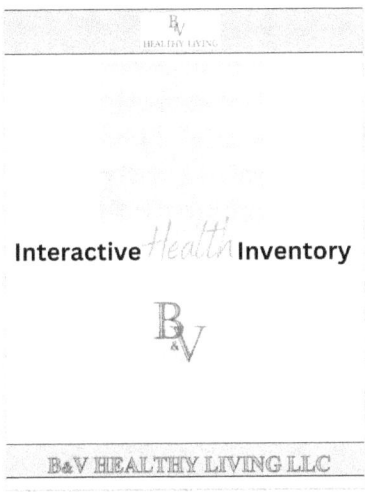

A FREE GIFT TO OUR READERS
Download and print the **Two Pillars of Power:**
Interactive Health Inventory

The Health Inventory should be used as you progress through each chapter assessing your current health and setting new goals that will transform your life right away!
Visit the link:

https://bvhealthyliving.org/HealthInventory

INTRODUCTION

When you think of the two pillars, picture them as two narrow columns of stone, like those of the ancient temples in Greece, still standing today after thousands of years of war and weather. Imagine you stand atop them, with a foot planted on each. When the pillars are weak, they are prone to breaking, falling, and swaying at the slightest hurricane of life. If one sways or topples, you'll be left flailing, likely to fall, and no matter how strong the other is, it cannot hold you alone. When they are both strong, they will support you through your decisions, pursuits, and adventures, and you can pursue your dreams and goals with surety, knowing you have a solid foundation for growth. So, what are the two pillars?

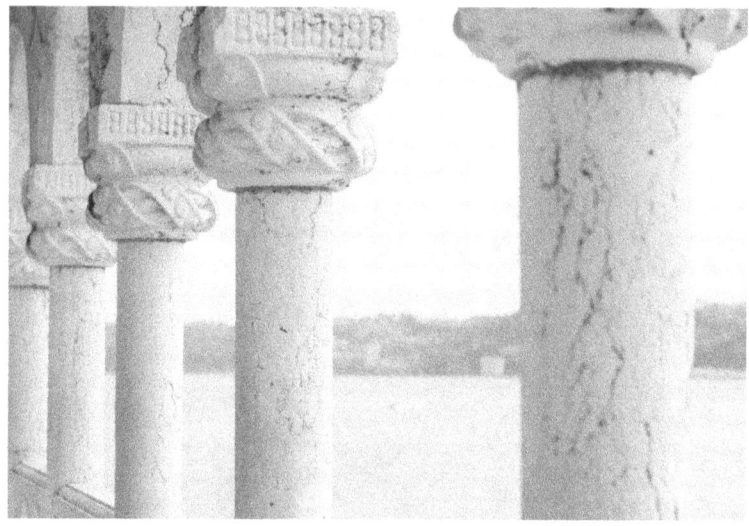

Mental and physical health are the two columns upon which your whole life depends. The deep-rooted connection between them has the power to alter your life for both good and bad. Your mental health and mind are the power behind focus, effort, ambition, and emotion, while your physical health and body are the tools that allow you to pursue adventure and the milestones of life. Both require great care and attention to live up to their full potential and provide optimal support throughout your life. The connection between them runs deep in our cells, nerves, hormones, and chemicals, rippling through our bodies in our blood. When one suffers, the other suffers too—a healthy body requires a healthy mind, and vice versa. Perhaps this has brought you to this book. You can feel that your pillars are imbalanced, that you are flailing and in need of support. You recognize that something about how you have been living your life isn't working in the best interests of your health, ambitions, or happiness, and you are looking to change that. This is the first, all-important step in the journey to come. Finding the energy and motivation to make the change you need in life.

This catalyst for change comes when you cannot stand the idea of going on the way you have been when you believe you deserve better. Many people struggle with mental health to the point they cannot leave the house, keep a job, sustain a healthy diet, or cannot form healthy relationships. People with physical health issues can find they have no energy or ability to socialize, work, clean, or exercise. Alongside pain and illness, they can easily develop mental health problems. In almost every success story, there has been a moment of clarity about the situation, an overwhelming desire to make positive change, and a need to break the negative cycle and take back control of life and health. This is that point.

This is the beginning of your success story, and like the others who have succeeded, you will turn your life around and find purpose, joy, health, and vitality again. With this book, you can rebuild your life, pursue your dreams and ambitions, and feel energized and healthy, well-rested and focused. You can get up and face the world, take control of your future, and forge a path of positivity.

Of course, lasting and positive change doesn't happen overnight. It takes dedication and discipline every day to rein in your life and take back control of it, to undo the bad habits and routines, to dispel the doubts and distractions, but with this book as your guide, you have the opportunity to make an incredible difference to your life in just a week. You'll be given an in-depth understanding of the two pillars of mental and physical health, plus information and exercises on eating right for your body, finding time for fitness, encouraging replenishing sleep, overcoming mental health roadblocks, building good habits and routines, and much more. Interactive activities will help you to focus your efforts and self-reflect on your needs and progress, and by the end of the book, you will have learned skills and built habits that you can harness to change your life in just one supercharged week. That incredible week starts right now, from the moment you turn this page and begin your journey to a fulfilling and happy life. Let's get started!

1

THE TWO PILLARS: A PERFECT PARTNERSHIP

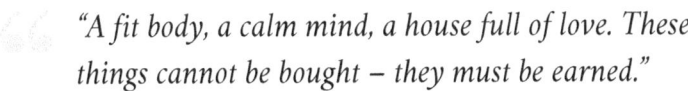

"A fit body, a calm mind, a house full of love. These things cannot be bought – they must be earned."

— NAVAL RAVIKANT

The key to a perfect partnership is balance, mutual support, and an understanding of each person's pivotal role in the partnership—the same is valid for mental and physical health. Everyone strives to be happy and healthy in mind and body. Still, without understanding the deep connection between the two pillars, it is easy to fall into habits that favor one or the other and, in doing so, unbalance everything. An awareness of how your mental and physical health intertwines will encourage you to make informed and effective choices about your health and help you to view yourself with empathy and your problems with clarity.

WHAT IS MENTAL HEALTH?

Mental health encompasses our emotional and psychological states, as well as our personal and social well-being. It plays a vital part in how we act, react, think, feel, and approach the world, from solving problems and dealing with stress, conflict, and emotions to showing empathy for and understanding others. Mental health influences our thoughts and actions throughout our lives, and it constantly changes and evolves as we experience and learn more about ourselves and the world. A healthy mind with a positive mindset is vital to enjoying life, being successful in your endeavors, supercharging your self-confidence, and achieving your goals, while poor mental health can prevent you from pursuing your ambitions and reaching your full potential—this is why mental health is one of the two vital pillars of life. Struggling with mental health is nothing to be ashamed of—almost everyone you meet is struggling in some way—but by recognizing the negative impact it can have on your life and working to take back control of your mind to find purpose and happiness again, is the most extraordinary act of kindness you can do yourself.

Factors That Impact Mental Health

Our minds are complex and advanced, and every single decision you make, and everything that happens to you has an impact on you and your mental health. Some experiences will strengthen, others may harm, and you must find ways to maintain a positive mindset to progress through life. Someone in a state of good, strong mental health is better equipped to face challenges and form connections than someone who is struggling with theirs, which highlights the importance of working to improve your mindset. There are many factors that contribute to mental health problems, almost all of which are negative experiences forced on us throughout our lives that damage our sense of self and self-worth and force us to question or relinquish control over our lives. These factors include isolation and loneliness, childhood abuse and neglect, trauma, discrimination, bullying, domestic violence, and grief, all of which can have lasting impacts on children and adults. Economic disadvantages like unemployment, poverty, debt, and homelessness also damage our mental health, as does severe or long-term stress and addiction.

Lifestyle factors such as diet, lack of sleep, work, and drugs can also lead to struggles with mental health, although more often, they are part of a more significant problem. While you should seek professional help and treatment for mental health problems, it is also essential to rule out any potential physical causes first to ensure you get the help you really need.

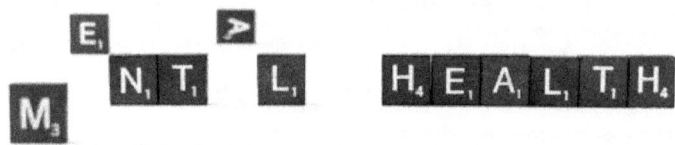

Mental Health Disorders

Mental health disorders and illnesses are more common than many people realize. In the United States, it is estimated that more than one in five adults are living with mental illnesses of some kind, including behavioral and emotional disorders (National Institute of Mental Health, 2023). Millions of people live every day with any number or variety of mental disorders, from manageable to severe, and understanding the different and most common types will help you to recognize them in yourself and in others, meaning you can better understand yourself and your needs, and practice empathy with others.

Anxiety

There are multiple forms of anxiety, none of which is just feeling scared. Anxiety can be far more debilitating than the short bursts of fear and nervousness we are supposed to feel in times of stress. Instead, people with anxiety experience excessive and prolonged fear and worry, often without an obvious or immediate cause, which can seriously impact their everyday functioning. People can experience anxiety throughout their lives, from childhood to adulthood, and can struggle to make friends, progress in education and employment, and form healthy relationships. Some of the many varieties of anxiety are general anxiety disorder, panic disorder, social anxiety, and separation anxiety.

Depression

Depression, a common and severe mental disorder, is characterized by long-term feelings of sadness, emptiness, and irritability, often combined with a lack of energy and interest, loss of pleasure in things, poor concentration and memory, feeling guilty, worthless, or hopeless, and experiencing suicidal or morbid thoughts. Physically, a depressed person may feel constantly tired, have trouble sleeping, experience weight and appetite fluctuations, and frequent headaches and pains. There are effective treatments available for depression, including psychotherapy and, in some instances, medication.

Bipolar Disorder

This mental disorder causes alternating mood, activity, and energy shifts, switching between depressive and manic episodes. Symptoms include "up" periods of feeling elated, impulsive, highly energized, and irritable to "down" periods of indifference, hopelessness, and other depressive behavior. These episodes can last days or weeks at a time and tend to go through cycles. Long-term treatment is usually necessary to manage bipolar disorders.

PTSD

Post Traumatic Stress Disorder manifests after exposure to a traumatic event that is often horrific and threatening. PTSD is most often characterized by re-living the event (in flashbacks, nightmares, and intrusive memories), avoiding thoughts, memories, people, and situations that remind the sufferer of the event, and experiencing persistent feelings of threat. Symptoms can last from weeks up to years and have a catastrophic impact on daily life—luckily, there are effective psychological treatment options.

Schizophrenia

This serious disorder affects how a person feels, thinks, behaves, and perceives the world. Symptoms include psychotic episodes with hallucinations, delusions, and noticeable thought and movement disorders. Other symptoms can appear similar to depression and other mental illnesses, like struggling to concentrate, plan, or take interest, and trouble with memory and decision-making. People with schizophrenia are not often violent to others. Still, they can be a danger to themselves, and treatment is essential to help them manage the condition and improve their ability to function in daily life.

Eating Disorders

The most common eating disorders are anorexia, bulimia, and binge-eating disorder. These are not simply diet or lifestyle choices. They are serious illnesses that impact behavior, thought, and emotions and harm the body. People suffering from anorexia and bulimia may avoid or severely restrict food, weigh themselves frequently or obsessively, and be unable to see themselves as anything other than "overweight" no matter how they look. They may purge food by vomiting, exercise excessively, and even use laxatives. Binge-eating disorder is characterized by a loss of control over eating. The person may consume large amounts of food in short periods of time, eat when they're not hungry, feel guilty or ashamed about eating, and hide food to eat in secret. They are likely to be overweight or obese and struggle to lose weight even when dieting. Eating disorders can be managed and treated with psychotherapy and medication.

Disruptive Behavior and Dissocial Disorders

Symptoms of these disorders usually, but not always, manifest in childhood and include persistent problems with behavior, defiance, disobedience, and conduct that violates others' fundamental rights and societal norms and rules. Treatment usually involves parents and teachers and cognitive and social skills training.

Neurodevelopmental Disorders

Neurodevelopmental Disorders develop during childhood and adolescence and affect cognitive and behavioral development, often resulting in problems with motor skills, language and understanding, and social skills. There is a wide range of disorders in this area, some very manageable, others more serious. Some common ones are Attention Deficit Hyperactivity Disorder (ADHD), autism spectrum disorder, and intellectual development disorders.

WHAT IS PHYSICAL HEALTH?

Maintaining good physical health is crucial for your well-being, quality of life, and your view of yourself. Physical health encompasses your fitness level and your body's ability to fight disease and work at peak function to support you through life. There are many benefits to having good physical health, including having more energy, living longer, being better equipped to fight illness, getting a better night's sleep, and being able to enjoy active pursuits. For many people, having good physical health enables them to feel strong and confident in their body and gives them peace of mind knowing they look after themselves. Working to strengthen your body and care for yourself also helps you better understand your body and its needs so you can recognize the symptoms and warning signs of disease earlier.

Factors That Impact Physical Health

As with mental health, there are many external and internal factors that affect our physical health and our ability to look after ourselves. You have control over some elements, like diet, lifestyle, and physical activity, whereas you cannot control others, like age and genetics. Lifestyle choices such as diet, exercise, and what you eat and drink and put into your body (including alcohol and smoking) have a powerful effect on the body, as do environmental factors like sun exposure or proximity to harmful substances. Your human biology (genetics and physiology) plays a crucial part, with factors making it easier or harder to maintain and achieve good physical health. Access to good healthcare is another vital factor, and regular check-ups and quick treatments can substantially impact your body's health.

Physical Health Disorders

The body is very complex and, as such, finds itself vulnerable to illnesses and diseases at every stage of life, no matter how healthy or careful you are. Unlike mental health disorders, physical disorders can be evident and have a noticeable impact on your daily life. While keeping healthy can prevent illnesses from causing long-term damage or even death, it is always best to be aware of the dangers and symptoms of some common physical health disorders. Hence, you are able to recognize them quickly and understand the problem. Symptoms can appear suddenly or grow slowly over time, so frequent check-ups can be instrumental, especially if you have a family history of medical conditions.

Cancer

One of the most common health conditions in the world, cancer occurs when cells grow uncontrollably and spread to areas of the body where they don't belong. There are many forms of cancer as these cells can and will grow anywhere in the body, but some of the most prevalent cancers are lung, breast, skin, prostate, and stomach. While cancer can be frightening, the earlier it is diagnosed, the better, and more treatments are available than ever.

Respiratory Diseases

Illnesses and disorders like asthma, bronchitis, pneumonia, chronic obstructive pulmonary disease (COPD), and cystic fibrosis cause breathing difficulties and chest pain. They can put a strain on the heart and muscles due to a lack of oxygen. They are usually treated with medication.

Diabetes

There are two types of diabetes. The most common, Type 2, is characterized by the body being unable to produce enough insulin, while Type 1 is a lifelong condition in which the immune system attacks insulin-producing cells. People that have Type 2 diabetes can reduce the risk and effects of it with medication and lifestyle changes like healthy eating and regular exercise. In contrast, Type 1 can only be treated with medication. Diabetes can cause high blood pressure, kidney disease, heart disease, and even sight loss.

Arthritis

Arthritis is a long-term condition, often occurring later in life (though not always), in which joints become swollen, stiff, and painful, making physical activity uncomfortable or difficult. It primarily affects the spine, knees, hips, and hands. There are many types of arthritis, including rheumatoid, osteoarthritis, gout, and fibromyalgia, so getting an accurate diagnosis is essential if you start to notice symptoms since each is treated differently. Treatments to reduce swelling can slow the progress of arthritis, while surgery and pain management are long-term options.

Osteoporosis

This condition weakens the bones causing them to become brittle and more likely to fracture and break. It can take years to develop and is often only diagnosed once a break has occurred, most often in the hips, spine, or wrists due to a fall. Osteoporosis is common in older people, and women are particularly prone to it after menopause. The only treatments are avoidance—avoiding breakages as much as possible—and taking bone-strengthening medication.

Obesity

Obesity, or carrying excessive body fat, is a serious medical condition with many associated health risks, including stroke, cancer, heart disease, and type 2 diabetes. It also negatively impacts mental health and quality of life. While over-eating foods with high-fat content are prime causes of obesity, there can also be medical and genetic reasons, such as an underactive thyroid gland or taking steroids. Obesity can be treated with regular exercise and a reduced-calorie diet, though medication or surgery may be necessary in some extreme cases.

Chronic pain

Chronic pain is persistent pain lasting for weeks or months, usually caused by an injury or operation, although it can also appear in times of increased stress or unhappiness. Sufferers can subside the pain with medication and applied heat, but physical therapy, lifestyle changes, exercise, and even psychotherapy can be very effective for long-term relief.

Neurological disorders

These are conditions that affect the nerves, brain, and spinal cord, caused by abnormalities in the nervous system. There are many different neurological disorders, including epilepsy and seizures, Alzheimer's disease and dementia, Parkinson's disease, and strokes. They are all complex conditions with specialized treatments and varying symptoms, though, for many, the risk grows with age. Genetic and environmental factors most often cause them, though injury, drug use, and brain infections can cause epilepsy and seizures too.

Infectious diseases

We've all had cold and flu at some point—often multiple times a year—but there are many infectious diseases out there that we are at risk of catching without warning, such as hepatitis, Lyme disease, measles, stomach flu, sexually transmitted infections, HIV/AIDS, and tuberculosis. These diseases can be caused by bacteria, fungi, parasites, viruses, or through direct contact transmission, food contamination, or bites. Symptoms can include prolonged fever, fatigue, coughing, diarrhea, and severe headaches, and it is best to get a doctor's diagnosis so you can receive the proper treatment. You can prevent most infectious diseases by getting vaccinations, preparing food safely, washing hands regularly, and practicing safe sex.

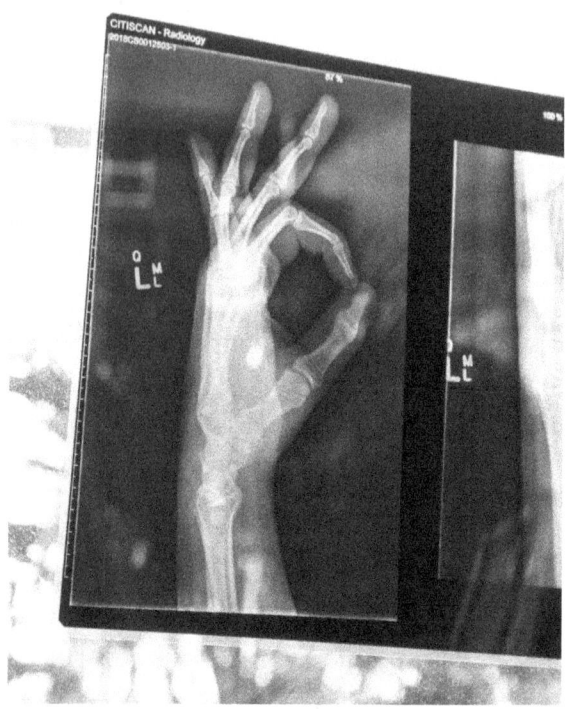

THE MENTAL AND PHYSICAL CONNECTION

Since mental and physical health are intrinsically linked, both significantly impact the other. The risk of developing a mental health problem is increased considerably by physical health problems, and vice versa. People suffering from physical health conditions may experience long-term pain and a loss of control over their body, which can lead to depression, anxiety, and low self-esteem, and those with serious health problems can also become isolated by their illnesses, unable to play an active part in society and maintain healthy relationships. When you are unable to exercise and socialize, you can quickly fall into negative thinking patterns and feel trapped, lonely, and hopeless. If your physical health increases fatigue, you are more likely to feel despondent and struggle to find the energy to socialize even more. Sometimes physical disorders lead to weight changes, skin conditions, and hair loss, which can have a negative impact on self-image. Being diagnosed with certain illnesses, particularly ones like cancer or HIV/AIDS, is enough to cause anxiety and stress and lead to depression.

Personal experience has proven to us how quickly one pillar can start to crack and weaken when the other pillar begins to crumble. Just this year, one of your authors experienced an injury that rapidly diminished their physical health, leading to a plummet in their mental health just as quickly. We have first-hand proof of how something as small and insignificant as a broken big toe can drastically impact your life. Excruciating pain, and a walking boot, meant no physical exercise or activities for several months. The first pillar breaks. This led to prompt weight gain that caused a tremendous negative impact on your author mentally. Depression and anxiety began to set in. The second pillar began to crumble. The injury took nearly seven months to heal (well enough) to resume a regular exercise routine, getting the author back to their original weight and improving their mental health. The physical health pillar was standing again, and the mental health pillar was starting to rebuild. We fully understand the power of the two pillars working in unison.

The brain plays one of the most vital roles in our bodies, so when our mental health suffers, it also directly impacts the body. If the brain cannot function healthily, neither can the body. Mental health problems can be linked to physical symptoms like headaches, fatigue, stomach and digestive issues, heart disease, and respiratory problems. They can also lead to insomnia and sleep apnea—which have a noticeably negative effect on the body—and difficulty concentrating, which can increase stress. Those suffering from mental health problems are also more likely to turn to smoking, drinking, and occasionally drugs to help them cope, and all of these come with severe and significant physical health impacts, including cancer, heart disease, and addiction. Adverse mental health has the ripple effect of making us feel less energized, so exercising routinely becomes a struggle, making us more likely to develop unhealthy eating habits leading to obesity or eating disorders.

Yet, for all these negative connections, there are many positive ones! The power of the mind over the body, and the other way around, can be used to combat disorders and improve health and quality of life. Exercise is proven to reduce stress and elevate our moods, so both mind and body are positively impacted, and maintaining a healthy and enjoyable diet nourishes your body and mind equally. These lifestyle choices put you in control of your health, reduce the risk of physical injury and illness, and keep you focused, centered, and energized. In later chapters, we'll closely explore factors like exercise and diet to increase understanding and awareness of the positive power of the two pillars of mental and physical health over our lives.

INTERACTIVE ELEMENT: HEALTH INVENTORY

Now you have a deeper understanding of the factors that are involved in mental and physical health and the critical connection between the two. It's time to start your journey toward taking control of your life and health and wielding the power of mind and body to your advantage. We'll start with a health inventory, so you can understand where you are starting from and form a clear idea of where you would like to end up.

Go to **https://bvhealthyliving.org/HealthInventory** to receive your free copy of the Interactive Health Inventory automatically, if you haven't done so already. These questions will help you assess your current physical and mental health and start to pinpoint areas that need attention and improvement. Answer them honestly and openly, without judgment or guilt, and know they are for you only to help you take the following steps to a better life.

Your Mental and Physical Health Inventory

To begin, answer these questions to get a baseline for your health:

- Do you currently have any physical health disorders?
- Do you currently have a diagnosed mental health disorder?
- Do any of your close relatives have:

  - A heart condition?
  - Respiratory problems?
  - Diabetes or weight-related problems?

- Is there a family history of:

  - Addiction?
  - Cancer?
  - Mental health disorders?

Based on your answers, you can already see some of the major factors that can have an impact on your health. When a family history of illness is involved, it is best to get a full physical from a doctor and discuss the potential dangers to your own health from genetic diseases and disorders.

Now, it's time for the questionnaire! Answer honestly and without overthinking to get the most accurate results. The questions are divided into three sections—mental, physical, and nutritional health. For each question, answer on a scale of 1-5:

- 1 = Always
- 2 = Frequently
- 3 = Sometimes
- 4 = Rarely
- 5 = Never

MENTAL HEALTH

1. I find it easy and fulfilling to discuss my problems with others.
2. I don't bottle up my feelings.
3. I don't feel stressed or anxious every day.
4. I make time for myself or my hobbies every day.
5. I meet up with my friends or family every week.
6. I practice self-care or self-reflection at least once a week (e.g., journaling, pampering, meditation).

PHYSICAL HEALTH

7. I do vigorous cardio-based exercise (e.g., swimming or running) at least three times a week.
8. I do stretching or strengthening exercises (e.g., yoga, Pilates, or weight lifting) at least three times a week.
9. I sleep 7-9 hours every night.
10. I make time for an exercise-related hobby (e.g., hiking) every week.
11. When I am injured or unwell, I seek medical help and advice.
12. I practice monthly self-examinations for cancer.
13. I have dental check-ups twice a year.
14. I maintain a healthy weight for my age/height/body type etc.

NUTRITION

15. I eat a varied diet from a wide range of food groups.
16. I avoid ultra-processed foods, which are high in fat and sugar.
17. I eat breakfast.
18. I don't snack between meals.
19. I limit my consumption of alcohol to the recommended amount or less.

20. I cook meals rather than order takeout at least
six days a week.

Now, total up your score. Remember, whatever you score,
it's not too late to make positive changes to your lifestyle
and habits to improve your well-being.

- Less than 40: Great, you're on a good path to a
  healthy life!
- 41-60: You'll see some areas you can focus on
  improving.
- 61-80: Shows there are a number of areas that
  require your attention.
- 81-100: Indicates that you are struggling to lead a
  balanced and healthy life and need to make some
  significant changes.

Look at your answers and pay close attention to anything
rated 4 or 5. These are the areas where you need to focus
your efforts. Are there any patterns? Can you draw any
lines between issues? Are the issues mainly mental or
physical, or a fair mix of both? Did anything surprise you?
Was there any area you've been overlooking?

Based on your answers to the questionnaire and the questions above, take your time to write down 3-5 goals for
both mental and physical health to focus on throughout
this book. You might want to prioritize your diet or exercise, or maybe you need to focus on your mental health—

whatever you need, make a clear goal for yourself. If you can, set separate diet, exercise, and self-care goals, as throughout the book, we will look at each of these areas in-depth and find ways to make positive changes using these factors.

Now you have a clear picture of your health and have set some goals to focus your efforts on. In the next chapter, we'll take a deep dive into nutrition, one of the crucial factors of a healthy and balanced life.

2

NOURISHING YOURSELF THE RIGHT WAY

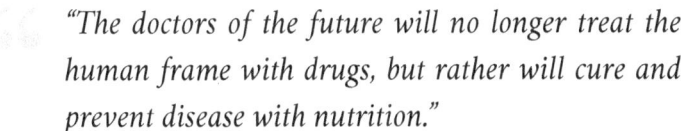

"The doctors of the future will no longer treat the human frame with drugs, but rather will cure and prevent disease with nutrition."

— THOMAS EDISON

T homas Edison was spot on when he said that quote because food is perhaps the most excellent medicine of all. Aside from being delicious—which immediately ranks it high above powdery pills and nauseating syrups—it is natural and accessible to all, full of the goodness of nature and all the essential nutrition the human needs. A nutritious diet is proven to have incredible health benefits, from increased energy levels and clearer skin to significantly boosted immunity and organ performance and reduced risk of serious disease. So, what are you waiting for? It's time to set aside the sweet treats, salty snacks, and takeout and start filling your body with the fabulous fuel of a nutritious and delicious diet.

WHAT IS NUTRITION?

Nutrition focuses on the relationship between our bodies and the combination of nutrients we put into them. Nutrients are the essential vitamins, minerals, and substances required to nourish and support the body in its health, healing, development, reproduction, and growth, and we get almost all of them exclusively from our food, which is why a nutritious diet is so crucial to living a healthy life. Eating a diverse and nutritious diet helps you to stay fit and energetic, your organs and cells to function optimally, and your body to fight infection and illness. It also improves mood and helps to curb bad eating habits like binging and snacking. While you may try to eat a balanced diet, good nutrition can be impacted by lifestyle and financial factors, and time constraints. For example, busy people often turn to microwave meals or takeout to get the energy they need as fast as possible. Still, these meals usually end up needing more nutrients, and you have no control over the ingredients. Taking control of your diet and what you put into your body is the first step toward a healthier life, and it's a straightforward one once you understand what good nutrition entails.

The Essential Nutrients

A balanced diet consists of regularly consuming essential nutrients across a variety of foods. The body itself cannot make these nutrients in large enough quantities, so we have to get them through our diet. There are two different categories of nutrients; macronutrients and micronutrients.

Macronutrients

Protein, fat, and carbohydrates are all macronutrients. Macronutrients need to be eaten in large amounts and form the main components of your diet.

Protein is used for growth, healing, and strength; all your hormones and antibodies are made of protein. The body uses protein to make amino acids, which are vital for survival. Meat, fish, and eggs are high in protein, and, luckily for vegetarians and vegans, so are beans, nuts, soy, and some grains.

Carbohydrates are your primary energy source, fueling your brain and nervous system and boosting the immune system. 45-65% of your daily calories should come from carbohydrates. While low-carb diets have taken over the world, there's no reason to avoid them. Healthy carbohydrates like whole grain pasta and bread, high-fiber fruit and vegetables, and beans are an excellent alternative to refined grains, white bread, and foods with added sugar.

Fats are crucial for vital bodily functions like vitamin and mineral absorption, cell building, blood clotting, and muscle movement. While it is high in calories and often viewed as unhealthy, these calories are an essential source of energy and not to be drastically limited. Healthy, unsaturated fats are found in nuts, seeds, vegetable oils, and fish. These fats balance blood sugar—helping to prevent type 2 diabetes and heart disease—and reduce inflammation, lowering the risk of cancer and arthritis. It would be best to limit trans fats and animal-based saturated fats like butter, cheese, and red meat from your diet.

Micronutrients

Vitamins and minerals are the two branches of micronutrients. They both support the body's vital functions and are essential to a healthy diet and body. They are found in all food groups and are particularly rich in fruit, vegetables, nuts, and seeds.

Each of the 13 essential vitamins has an important part to play in the body and needs to be consumed regularly in the proper amounts for the body to function optimally. Many adults do not get enough vitamins, but they are easy to get if you eat a wide-ranging diet full of fruit and vegetables. Vitamins are antioxidants that are crucial for maintaining healthy skin, bones, and vision. They also boost the immune system, helping protect and heal the body, and they can lower the risk of some cancers.

Minerals, like iron, zinc, and calcium, are essential for many bodily functions, for example, hydration, strengthening bones and teeth, regulating metabolism and blood pressure, healing, and hormone creation.

Water

Water is crucial, and not only because it makes up over 60% of the human body. Water has many incredible effects on the body, acting as a shock absorber, lubricating joints, flushing out toxins, carrying nutrients through the body, hydrating, and promoting healthy digestion. It is also proven to improve brain function.

THE DANGERS OF DIET CULTURE

Diet culture has become a disturbingly prevalent part of society, with increasing pressure on people to aspire to certain body types, appearances, and lifestyles, often with an emphasis on food restriction, obsessive exercising, and avoiding "fatness" leading to overwhelming anxiety about failing to meet society's aesthetic and the consequences that will have on your life. Many of the diets and lifestyles we see on social media are unsuitable or attainable. Still, nevertheless, we try to adhere to them, often causing financial, physical, and emotional problems. Diet culture sets high, often impossible, standards for our bodies, and when you fail to attain or maintain the desired physical outcome, it can lead to shame, guilt, negative self-image, and a sense of failure. It also encourages negative, restrictive, and compulsive eating and exercising behaviors, which means things you should enjoy become punishing and unenjoyable.

Diet culture also skews our sense of worth, telling us that in order to be accepted and admired in society, you must meet specific physical standards regardless of your age, sex, body type, financial situation, and mental and physical health factors. It is essential to understand that health is not based on size or weight and that each of us has a different metabolism and body structure which means diet and exercise are different for everybody. An obsession with body image can have many negative impacts, including malnutrition and dehydration, constipation, mood swings, poor sleep quality, cardiovascular problems, muscle loss, and eating disorders.

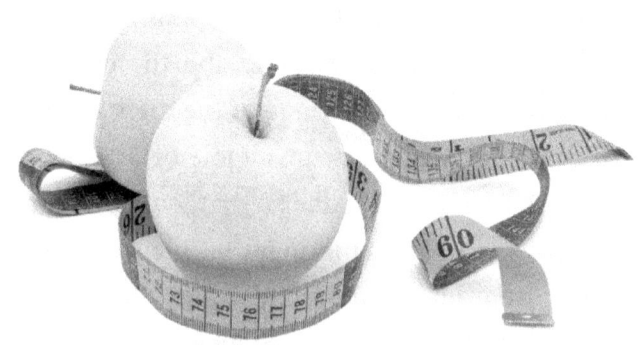

Symptoms of Disordered Eating

Eating disorders can appear gradually and be hard to spot, especially for the sufferer, so knowing the symptoms to look out for could be vital to helping yourself or someone else recognize when they are in danger. While eating disorders can be treated with mental and physical care, catching them as early as possible significantly increases the chances of recovery and decreases the long-term effects on the body and mind. Symptoms of disordered eating include:

- Preoccupation or obsession with weight, food, dieting, and calorie counting.
- Refusal to eat certain types of foods or food groups, especially carbohydrates and fats.
- Skipping meals or severely limiting portion sizes.
- Noticeable emaciation, especially gaunt cheeks and collarbones.
- Social withdrawal and avoiding social activities where food is present.
- Trips to the bathroom right after meals.
- Extreme concern about physical appearance— they may check mirrors constantly and seek positive reinforcement about their body.
- Changes or irregularities in the menstrual cycle.
- Difficulty concentrating and mood swings.
- Dizziness, fainting, and insomnia.

- Dental problems, including cavities, discoloration of teeth, and sensitive teeth.
- Poor immunity leads to slower wound healing and frequent illness.
- Dry skin and hair.
- Cuts and callouses on finger joints.
- Feeling cold all the time and blotching on the hands and feet.

By remembering that all our bodies are unique and have different needs, we can see the futility of diet culture. Instead, it is best to focus on building a healthy and nutritious diet and lifestyle based on moderation of food and understanding our bodies. For help with unhealthy eating habits, it is best to see a professional nutritionist or dietician and ignore social media entirely. After all, food should be delicious, enjoyable, satisfying, and nourishing, and should be allowed to be one of the great pleasures of our lives!

HOW DIET IMPACTS HEALTH

Physical Impact

The physical impacts of poor nutrition can be extreme and detrimental to normal bodily function. They can tremendously increase the risk of obesity, type 2 diabetes, heart disease, high blood pressure, cancer, and high cholesterol. With poor nutrition comes fatigue and poor brain function, including a lack of concentration and trouble with memory, and a noticeable loss of energy, stamina, and strength, making exercise more difficult and further aggravating the problem. The immune system is seriously impacted by poor nutrition, which causes frequent and more prolonged illnesses and difficulty healing wounds. Inflammation and oxidative stress increase, causing pain, anxiety, and even depression.

Mental Impact

A nourishing diet can also have repercussions on our mental health. Many foods promote a healthier mind, including green leafy vegetables, fatty fish, and berries. Nutrient-dense foods produce good gut bacteria that promote dopamine and serotonin production, which makes us feel happier. Foods that make us feel energized and focused, like whole grains and natural sugars, are remarkable for our mental health. In contrast, refined sugars and processed foods can cause inflammation, mood swings, and sugar crashes that negatively impact our brains. People struggling with mental health disorders are likely to have poor nutrition because they make unhealthy food choices that do not offer the body what it needs--they may skip meals, choose fast and easy options like takeout or frozen meals, or they may develop cravings or food obsessions that cause them to only eat one type of food for long periods of time. They may also turn to alcohol to boost their mood, which means adding toxins to their diet. Fatigue and insomnia caused by poor diet can also lead to mental health problems like depression and anxiety.

STEPS TO IMPROVING YOUR DIET

Over our 20 years of marriage, we have had our peaks and valleys regarding nutrition and health. Vanda came to the United States with her European approach to the pure and clean eating habits she was raised on. You can imagine the shock to her system when she met her fast-food-loving husband. She swiftly adapted to the American culture's quick and easy eating habits, and Marshmallow Fluff and Oreo cookies became her comfort food of choice. As we began to expand our family, we also started to expand our waste lines. Careers, college courses, and small children were the catalysts for quick dinner options made of processed foods and zero time for outdoor activities and physical exercise. We have endured our share of physical health problems over the years, such as high blood pressure, high cholesterol, sleep apnea, and vertigo. We came to the realization that we needed to make significant changes in our lives if we wanted to live a healthier, happier, and longer life with our family. It all started with improving our diet.

Improving your diet doesn't mean making sudden and extreme changes but introducing healthier eating habits over time—you're more likely to keep a healthy diet if it isn't restrictive or hyper-controlled. Building good eating and cooking habits is the best way to maintain a nutritious diet, and it can take a little extra effort. It is worth it for the long-term physical and psychological benefits. Here are some steps to improve your diet that you can enact immediately:

- Eat breakfast every morning! Breakfast is the most important meal of the day, jump-starting your body with a dose of energy and sustenance so you can feel alert and ready to work and your organs wake up and start functioning. Whole grain cereal or toast, oatmeal, yogurt, fruit, and eggs are all great breakfast options.
- Stay hydrated by drinking water throughout the day, not just when you feel thirsty. If it helps, set a water reminder on your phone to go off every hour or so.
- Eat at least five portions of fruit and vegetables. We've all been told this for years now, but it still stands! The fruit and vegetables can be fresh, frozen, or dried, and smoothies and juice count too, so there are many ways to meet this target easily. A fun way to incorporate more vegetables and exercise is to go for a walk and visit your local farmers market! Vanda loves to grow her own vegetables in her garden as well. Nothing is more

satisfying than the smell and taste of a fresh
vegetable you grow yourself!

- One-third of your food should be starchy, high-
energy carbohydrates like pasta, rice, potatoes,
and bread—try to choose wholegrain options
whenever possible.

- Aim to eat at least two portions of fish every
week, one oily, like salmon or mackerel, and one
meaty, like cod or haddock. Fresh or frozen are all
great, though do be careful of smoked fish due to
its high salt content.

- Limit your saturated fat and sugar intake.
Saturated fat increases cholesterol, and sugar
contributes to weight gain, strokes, cancers, and
tooth decay and can cause erectile dysfunction!
Packaged and processed food and drinks contain
both of these, often in high quantities, so read
labels carefully.

- Keep your salt intake to no more than six grams
per day—a lot of our salt intake is in the food we
buy, so check for low-salt options and avoid
adding extra salt to food when cooking and
eating.

- Avoid snacking between meals—if you get hungry,
have some fruit or a protein bar, but nothing
heavy or processed.

- Limit yourself to two caffeinated drinks daily and
none after 6 p.m.

- Find ways to make your favorite meals healthier too. For example, use less oil for frying, swap meat for tofu or vegetables, or create your own sauces rather than store-bought ones. You can even make healthier pancakes with wholewheat flour and low-fat milk, and homemade pizza is easy to make and much more nutritious. We have had many fun family nights making homemade pizza with our children!

These are small but very effective changes you can make starting today. In the next section, we'll take a closer look at your eating habits and develop a plan to reach your nutrition goal.

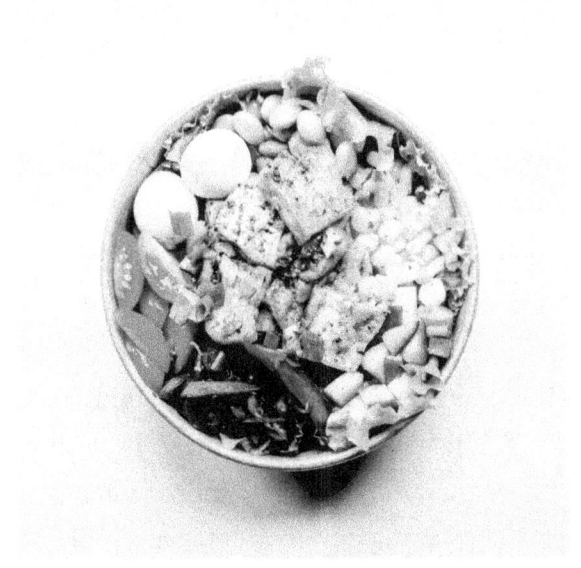

INTERACTIVE ELEMENT: EVALUATE YOUR EATING HABITS

Write down in your Health Inventory what you eat and drink on average each day of a typical week. Write down any snacks, drinks, meals, takeout, and any time you eat out, even if you get popcorn at the movie theatre. Take your time and be honest.

Now, looking at the list, look at it in terms of nutrition:

- Are all the food groups and essential nutrients represented?
- Are your meals balanced and full of vegetables?
- Can you count your five fruit and vegetables a day, every day?
- Are your snacks healthy?
- Do you cook from scratch more than you order in or have a frozen dinner?
- How much water do you drink in relation to caffeinated drinks and alcohol?
- Can you pinpoint any habits that could be considered diet culture habits?

Answer these questions by clearly identifying where your diet lacks nutrition. Remember, there is nothing to be ashamed of—you're on a path to improvement, and that's all that matters. From your answers, you should be able to see areas you can change your diet to make it more nutritious. Here are some easy ways you can make immediate and healthy changes to your eating habits:

- Write a daily meal plan for next week. From that plan, you can make a shopping list, pick up everything you need in advance, and be ready to start next week's nutrition journey! Meal plans are an excellent tool as they cut down on snacking and impulsive buying of food, and you know what you'll be eating, so you don't have to waste time and energy coming up with dinners every day. It also gives you control over your eating, ensuring you get what you need.

- Put a "no-buy" in place on the food you know is having a negative impact on your health. It can be for a couple of weeks or a month but stick with it and see how differently you feel afterward!

- Pay attention to portion sizes! People often overestimate how much food they actually need to eat in a meal. Food should leave you feeling energized, not stuffed. Weighing carbohydrates to ensure you get the recommended amount on your plate helps.

- Slow down when you eat! Try to take around 20 minutes to eat a main meal, and chew everything well. Also, try eating all your vegetables *first* to ensure you have room for them.

- Schedule meat-free days every week—just two days of vegetarian eating can make a massive difference to your energy levels and digestion.
- Try to eat a different dinner every day unless you're making use of leftovers—even then, spruce up those leftovers!
- Make simple but effective changes to your meals by swapping out bad for good! For example, swap fries for a baked potato or rice, white bread for wholegrain, deep-dish pizza for thin crust, chips for popcorn, sugary soda for sparkling water, and chocolate and sweets for dark chocolate, protein bars, or dried or fresh fruit. There are loads of great and easy swaps to make, so pick a few!

You can use your new knowledge of nutrition to work towards the fitness and health goal you set in the last chapter. The key to a healthy life is to commit to long-term changes rather than quick fixes, and the sooner you start, the better!

Now you're up to speed on nutrition and you've made positive changes to your diet, you'll soon feel more energized and in control of your body, so what better way to show it than to get your heart pounding and your muscles working? In the next chapter, we'll throw ourselves into exercise, one of the most important steps you can take to a stronger, healthier body and mind.

3

MOVING TOWARD HEALTH

> *"We cannot solve problems with the kind of thinking we employed when we came up with them."*
>
> — ALBERT EINSTEIN

The first few weeks of a new exercise regime are notoriously tough on the body and mind, and the struggle can be disheartening when you are forced to confront the truth about your fitness level. However, if you can push on and commit, the long-term rewards are worth persevering for! The key is finding a suitable exercise for your body, lifestyle, and needs. While some people are happy to hit the gym, others find it an intimidating and pressured environment and prefer to work out solo in the comfort of their homes. Lifting weights and toning up work for some, while others prefer swimming or running to make them feel stronger. Everyone is different, and when it comes to exercise, recognizing that difference can help you form a healthy and productive relationship with fitness. It's *never* too early or late to start working towards a healthier and stronger body, and you deserve to enjoy the benefits of an active life.

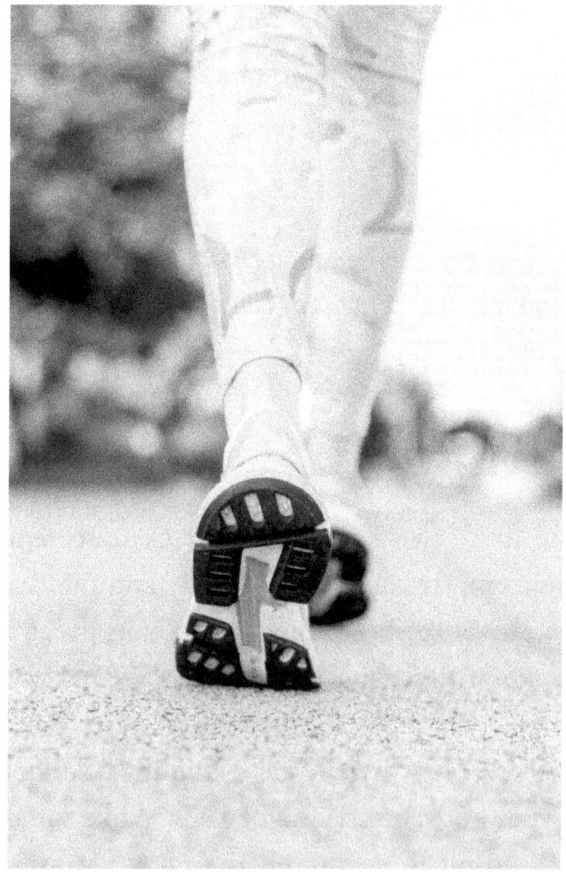

WHY DOES EXERCISE MATTER?

Exercise has a powerful effect on the body and mind—in fact, there are very few lifestyle choices that can make as significant, and as positive of an impact, as exercise! Engaging in regular physical activity is one of the best things you can do for your health, not only because it gets your heart pumping and your organs working but because of the numerous benefits it brings. Exercise is proven to strengthen bone and muscle, reduce disease risk, manage weight, and improve concentration, focus, and energy. Many adults find themselves in jobs or leisure time that involves extended periods of time sitting down, whether in an office or on your sofa, and all this sitting has a negative impact on the body. Notably, it can cause ergonomic issues that lead to weakened joints, bad—and painful— posture, weight gain, and fatigue. While you cannot change your working conditions, and while you should enjoy leisure time, you can choose to make time for some form of exercise every day, even if it is just taking a walk or stretching. Set an alarm to remind yourself to get up and move your body periodically during your day! There is a form of exercise for everyone, and everyone can experience the benefits of exercise, no matter their age, gender, lifestyle, ethnicity, genes, or size.

Most people's exercise journeys begin with a weight-loss goal, and while this is a commendable goal, it should not be the only reason to exercise! Even the fittest people, and those blessed with that elusive gene that means they never gain weight, should make room for exercise in their lives, and not just for aesthetic gain, but for their internal and mental health. Physically, regular exercise can reduce the risk of developing several cancers, type 2 diabetes, and cardiovascular diseases, and it can improve gut health, blood flow, and lung capacity. Although running and cardio exercises are popular, muscle-strengthening activities like weightlifting and yoga tone the body and protect the muscles from damage, while swimming, dancing, and Pilates are incredible full-body workouts. Finding exercises that work for you and your fitness goals and doing your research can also make a considerable impact—our bodies are all unique and need different attention, so if something works for someone else, be aware that it may not work for you, but something else always will!

The general rule is to aim to do at least 150 minutes of moderate physical activity every week. This can include walking, jogging, swimming, yoga or Pilates, or even dancing around the kitchen while dinner cooks, plus any number of other activities. One hundred fifty minutes sounds like a lot, right? It isn't! It works out to only 30 minutes five days a week, which really is a very manageable amount. You're probably thinking, "I have so much to do. Where will I find the time?" but it is infinitely worth carving out space in your day somehow, whether that means walking to work instead of driving, a morning jog, or a yoga session, a post-work swim (this is great, it really relaxes the body and settles the mind after a stressful day!), or a lunchtime walking session with your coworkers. Be the first to help inspire your team and build healthy habits together! As we'll discuss later in the chapter, there is always a way to incorporate exercise into your day, and even if you don't feel like doing it or you're tired, commit to it. Plug some of your favorite music into your ears that gets you going and inspired, and get your body moving! You'll discover you have more energy than you thought, and your body will thank you!

EXERCISE AND MENTAL HEALTH

If exercise works wonders for the body, that's nothing to what it can do for the mind! There is a magical quality to exercise. When you do it, your worries and cares fade away as your body takes over for a while, and your mind is free to relax and regroup. It's hard to worry about bills and the mortgage or get lost in dark thoughts when you're sweating your way through a Pilates session or counting reps at the gym. More than this, exercise causes the body to release "happy chemicals" like dopamine and serotonin that flood the body and noticeably boost your mood. Yet more beautiful effects are that it tires out your muscles so you sleep better and can wake more refreshed, and it increases your energy for the day by flooding the muscles (including the brain) with blood and oxygen. Also, exercise improves memory and thinking skills, contributing to an improved ability to handle stress. Partaking in exercise also removes the guilt of enjoying leisure time and food. In our modern society, productivity is the benchmark of success, so people often feel guilty for taking time out to rest and relax and instead find ways to mix leisure time with work time, for instance, by answering emails late into the night with only half an eye on the TV. If you've done exercise that day, you feel like you've accomplished something and find it easier to relax and enjoy food and time for yourself.

When it comes to mental disorders, exercise works its magic again. The increased sense of well-being it gives us reduces the symptoms of anxiety and depression and helps relieve symptoms of PTSD and trauma. In people with ADHD, it improves concentration and motivation. For people with eating disorders, exercise also improves self-esteem and gives you back control of your body. Exercise may not be able to cure these disorders, but it can go a long way to offering some much-needed relief from them.

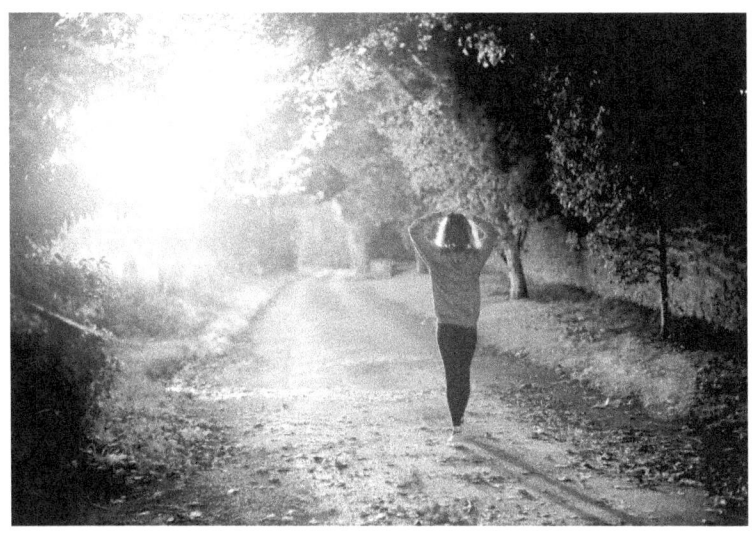

EXERCISING FOR BEGINNERS

Fitness Focus

Everyone's fitness journey starts somewhere, and the best way to start yours is by assessing your fitness level so you can make the right exercise choices and targets for your-self and your body's needs. Once you have a baseline, you can use it to measure your progress and see the incredible improvements you make in time.

Assess Your Fitness Level

You can assess your fitness level by yourself or ask someone to help you with the following activities. Remember not to judge yourself and simply do what you can—this is just the beginning of your journey, so you don't need to be perfect! Document your results in your Health Inventory checklist.

- Record your pulse rate before and after walking one mile (1.6 kilometers).
- Record how long it takes to walk 1 mile or run 1.5 miles (2.4 kilometers).
- Record how many push-ups you can do at a time.
- Record how far you can reach forward while seated on the floor with your legs outstretched in front of you—mark it on your leg with a pen to make measuring easier!
- Record your waist circumference.
- Record your body mass index (BMI).

Based on these results, you can set goals; for example, you may decide to shave 5 minutes off of your mile walk time within two weeks or improve your flexibility so you can touch your toes. Pick realistic goals and give yourself enough time to achieve them.

Design Your Fitness Program

Building your own fitness program is a great way to understand your body and goals, and also you can tailor it perfectly to suit your lifestyle, budget, and time constraints. Start by setting out your fitness goals clearly and realistically—remember that it takes time to build up fitness, so don't set goals and expect the achieve them in a week! Be honest with your abilities and the time available to you. You might have to move things around and prioritize, but keep your exercise consistent, as this will help it become part of your daily routine. Ensure that your exercise slots add up to 150 minutes of moderate exercise only or 75 minutes of intensive exercise a week, like HIIT training or dance classes—better yet, do a combination of both. Try to do some form of strength training for the whole body twice a week (yoga and Pilates are great if weights aren't your thing). Give yourself rest days; you'll need them!

Know Your Body

If you don't know where to start, your body will tell and show you where you need to focus your fitness efforts. Do you get out of breath quickly? Do your joints ache? Do you feel lethargic and struggle to get up in the morning? Do you have trouble lifting things? Does your dog drag you around the park more effortlessly than he used to? Take notice of your aches, pains, and physical limitations —these are the areas you should be working to improve.

Take a look at your body—not critically, not looking for flaws, but looking for areas you can tone, strengthen, and support. If you spend a lot of time at a desk, you might find your spine or shoulders are hunched, and your lower back is stiff. If you're on your feet all day, your knees and ankles may need strengthening. Find areas to work on but be kind to yourself!

Get Started!

The first steps of your exercise journey will seem like the toughest of all. Your body will ache, and your muscles will protest the new demands on them. You'll feel tired and unmotivated because progress will seem slow, but just start. The sooner you do, the sooner you can enjoy the benefits! Here are some tips for fitness beginners to help you through the first few difficult weeks:

- Start slow and low so you don't get overwhelmed, exhausted, intimidated, or worse, injured—little is better than none!
- Be sure to take the time to warm up and cool down before and after exercise—this helps to prevent injury and strain and makes the exercise itself easier.
- Be creative! Pick exercises that you enjoy or find inspiring, as you'll be more likely to stick with them. Combine nature and exercise if you can, such as hiking with friends.
- Be flexible. Not just physically, but with your time and plan. Unexpected things may throw it off, but don't let them derail the program. Instead, work around them and keep making time for exercise, even if it isn't what you planned for that day.
- Listen to your body.
- Ignore the mirror and the scale! You'll feel better in your body long before you see it, so it can be

disheartening if results aren't evident on the outside. Focus inwards and enjoy the feeling of change inside.

Monitor and Maintain

Monitor your progress by retaking the fitness test after six weeks, then six months, then a year (or as often as it makes you feel good), and you may notice you need to adjust your goals or routine. Health apps can be great for logging your exercise sessions so you can keep track of your active minutes and burned calories. If you notice you are struggling with the same exercise for a long time, or if your weight or size doesn't change steadily or at all, it is worth seeing if there is a medical reason for it.

FINDING TIME FOR FITNESS

In our busy world full of distractions, temptations, expectations, problems, and worries, it can seem like we already have so much on our plates that there's just no time for exercise. Our busy lives make us feel like we have to forgo fitness to face life's everyday challenges and errands, and when fitness starts to take a backseat, you pay the price. Here are some ways you can keep fitness in the foreground of your life and keep working towards your health goals.

- Capitalize on your commute. Consider running, walking, cycling, or jogging to work—or at least part of the way—if possible. Keep a change of clothes and some basic toiletries at work so you don't have to carry them with you.
- Keep workout clothes handy. By keeping workout clothes in your car or at the office at all times, you're equipped to switch into workout mode any time you have a spare 20 or 30 minutes.
- Run your errands—literally! Skip the car and walk, cycle, or run on your errands. This is a great way to get fresh air, exercise, and get everything done in one go, saving you time in the long run. If you must take a car to work or do errands, try parking as far away as possible to ensure you are at least gaining the most steps possible in your day.
- Schedule workouts as though they are meetings or appointments you can't miss—this will help you stick to them and prioritize them.
- Sweat while the kids are sweating! If your kids play sports or do activities, get a workout in while they're busy. You could run or walk around the field or park while they play or join in with them or the other parents.
- Get up earlier. Start your day just half an hour earlier to make time for exercise. This may be tough at first while your sleeping pattern adjusts, but a morning exercise session can help you feel

more energized and be more productive throughout the day.

- Find a gym close by. A conveniently placed gym that is quick and easy to get to will save you time on a busy day.
- Find a workout buddy! Working out with your partner or a friend can make exercise more enjoyable, social, and motivational, and you're less likely to skip a workout if it means letting someone else down.
- Keep a positive mindset. Don't let exercise become a chore that you just have to do—instead, find ways to keep it fun and exciting. Try new exercises and activities, get your friends or family involved whenever possible, and focus on the positives, like having more energy and a better relationship with your body when fitness gets tough.

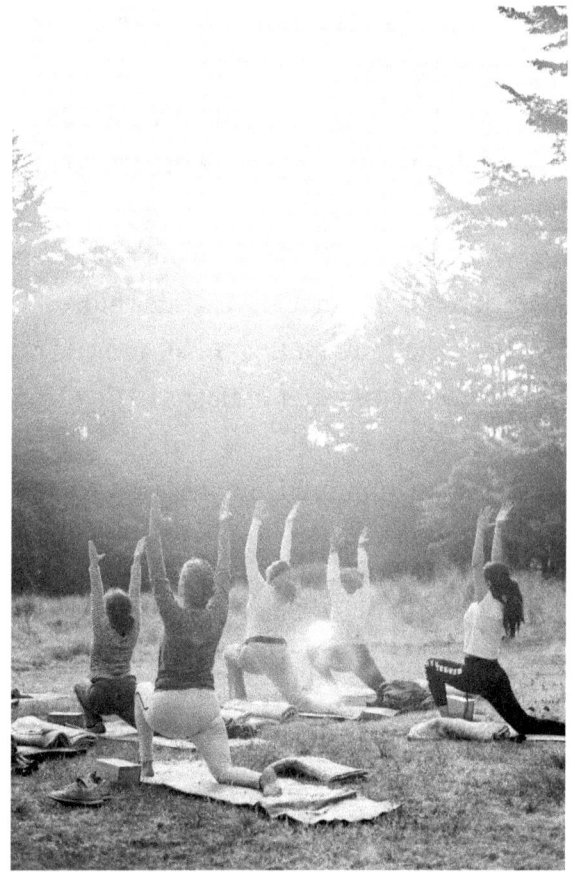

INTERACTIVE ELEMENT: EXERCISE CHART

In the Interactive Health Inventory, you will find an exercise chart like the one below, to help you log your fitness goals and progress and keep you on track to a fit and healthy you! Can you identify at least 3 opportunities throughout the day you can engage in exercise? There are opportunities even for the super busy individuals. Document a plan on the chart to stick to!

Finding Time for Fitness! Can you Exercise 3 times per day? (Target 150 min/moderate, or 75 min/intensive per week)	Results
6 AM 7 AM	• Are you able to wake up earlier? • Consider walking, running, jogging, cycling, or swimming to start your day more energized and be more productive throughout the day! • What can you try to implement? _____	___ Min ___ Min
8 AM	• Consider walking, running, jogging, or cycling to work. What a refreshing commute that can be! • What can you try to implement? _____	___ Min
9 AM 10 AM 11 AM	• Get up from that desk and walk more throughout the day! Drink more water and stay hydrated! • What can you implement? _____	___ Min ___ Min ___ Min
12 PM	• Can you go for a walk, or go to the gym on your lunch break? • What can you try to implement? _____	___ Min
1 PM 2 PM 3 PM 4 PM	• Get up from that desk and walk more throughout the day! Drink more water and stay hydrated! • What can you implement? _____	___ Min ___ Min ___ Min ___ Min
5 PM	• Consider walking, running, jogging, or cycling back home. What a refreshing commute that can be after a long day! • What can you try to implement? _____	___ Min
6 PM	• Run your errands...literally? Skip the car and walk, run, or cycle to your errands! • Gym after work? Running, jogging, cycling, or swimming? Sweat while the kids are sweating? • What can you try to implement? _____	___ Min

4

A RESTFUL APPROACH

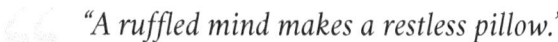 *"A ruffled mind makes a restless pillow."*

— CHARLOTTE BRONTË, ENGLISH NOVELIST
AND POET

Sleep is a crucial factor in our physical and mental well-being. In sleep, we rest our body and mind, heal, problem-solve, and reset, so we can wake up refreshed and energized for the day ahead. Those few magical hours of sleep are proven to have incredible effects on our mind and body, and you can definitely feel the difference in yourself and your energy levels after a good night's rest. It's ironic that in a busier and more demanding world than ever, we struggle more to sleep. We're exhausted by work and play, but our minds are so overstimulated by phones and so full of the anxieties of our lives that when our heads hit the pillow, sleep can often seem impossible. Night after night of disrupted or limited sleep, our worries and anxieties multiply further as our bodies protest and our minds become forgetful and easily distracted. Finding ways to encourage and ensure a good night's sleep is one of the most important steps you can take on your journey to a healthier body and mind.

THE SCIENCE OF SLEEP

In order to get a good night's sleep, you need to go through the four stages of sleep. Specific patterns in brain activity characterize each of these stages—these cycles and stages of sleep are known as sleep architecture. They are split into two categories: Rapid Eye Movement (REM) sleep and non-REM (NREM) sleep.

NREM Sleep

Three of the four stages of sleep fall into this category. **N1**, the first stage, comes when you have just fallen asleep. This short stage lasts only a few minutes, but it is easy to disrupt as the body is not fully relaxed, and the brain activity is still relatively high. **N2** follows; when the body temperature drops, the muscles relax, and breathing and heart rate start really slowing down. Then you get to **N3**, a deep sleep, when the body relaxes even further, and pulse and breath slow significantly. It is hard to wake someone from this stage of sleep. Now your body is in the perfect state to rest and recuperate—the muscles can heal, the blood can oxygenate gently, and all the physical strain of the day can melt away.

REM Sleep

With the body relaxed, the mind can let go too. REM sleep is the most crucial sleep stage for cognitive function—like memory, learning, and creativity—and for improved mental performance. In this stage, your brain dumps information, solves problems and experiences the most vivid dreams of the sleep cycle.

Are You Getting Enough Sleep?

Almost everyone will struggle to get enough sleep at some point in their life. It may be that you find it challenging to get to sleep in the first place, you frequently wake in the night, or you may struggle with a sleep disorder, like snoring or sleep apnea, that disrupts your breathing. Getting the recommended hours of sleep for your age group every night is essential to ensure your body and mind can function optimally the next day. Children require at least ten hours of sleep a night, while teenagers should get 8-10 hours. The recommended amount for adults is 7+ hours a night, and for people over 60, it is 7-9 hours. Of course, these are only guidelines, and you'll find your sleep hours vary depending on the season (in summer, it is light later and longer, so that can influence your body clock), temperature, day of the week, and your mental state—anxiety can play havoc with sleep! Let's examine the effect of sleep on our mental and physical health.

SLEEP AND HEALTH

Scientists are constantly conducting sleep studies to discover more about the vital link between sleep and health. Physically, sleep is your body's chance to turn all its energy to healing and recovery, which is why when we are ill or injured, we often feel drained, as our body needs sleep in order to nurture us. Relaxed muscles ease inflammation, pain, and injury, and in sleep, cells regenerate quicker.

The link between sleep and mental health is fascinating— sleep problems can be both a cause and effect of mental health problems, creating a vicious circle. A lack of REM sleep can impair the brain's ability to process emotional information and regulate mood, leading to an increased risk and progression of mental disorders. The fatigue and tension caused by an unhealthy sleep pattern can worsen anxiety and depression, and the prevalence of suicidal thoughts and behaviors is significantly increased by prolonged lack of sleep. Sleep disorders like Obstructive Sleep Apnea (OSA), in which pauses in breath reduce the body's oxygen levels, can disrupt sleep and are more common in people with psychiatric conditions. Insomnia is both a cause and consequence of many mental disorders, and the impact it has on our daily lives is incredible.

You are more prone to making mistakes, leading to anxiety and self-doubt; you may struggle to be creative, which can impact both your work and leisure; and you may feel enormous guilt and loneliness due to a lack of energy for social interaction. Essentially, while sleep won't cure mental health disorders, it goes a long way to helping keep them in check and reduce their negative impacts on your life.

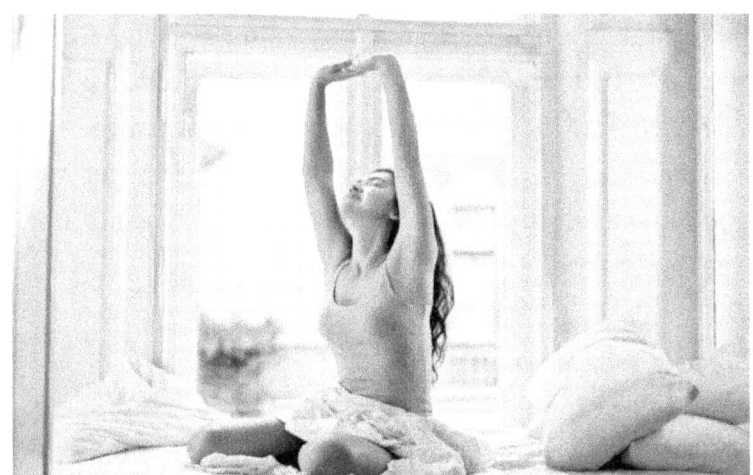

SLEEP HYGIENE

Sleep hygiene is the practice of keeping clean and healthy sleeping habits that help you to keep a positive and consistent sleep pattern and promote restful sleep. Good sleep hygiene is a simple yet effective way to improve your sleep quality dramatically. It helps you get to sleep faster, maintain sleep throughout the night and makes getting up in the morning easier. You'll feel more energized, focused, productive, and generally more positive in the morning. Building a stable sleep schedule is the principal aspect of sleep hygiene, as this gets your body into the routine of falling asleep quickly and like clockwork, rather than forcing it to stay awake or be unable to fall asleep when needed. Your sleep hygiene practices can be tailored to suit your lifestyle and needs, depending on your working hours, home and family situation, and any other time constraints. Whatever your circumstances, building a pre-bed routine and creating a sleeping environment that promotes quality deep sleep and reduces disruptions is the key to good sleep hygiene. In the next section, we'll look at ways to support yourself in getting a good night's sleep with some excellent sleep hygiene practices and habits.

Support Your Sleeping

You will need to change your environment and pre-sleep behavior in order to improve your sleep hygiene and sleep cycle. Making your bedroom the perfect place to sleep is a great way to begin.

Set the Scene for Sleep

Your bedroom should promote rest and relaxation, so start by keeping it clean and uncluttered—clutter can be distracting, and you want to avoid any mess that can cause odors and dust to build up. A fresh-smelling and clean room is not only healthier but also better for sleep. You can incorporate restful colors like blue, green, and orange into the decor, put dried lavender near the bed, burn relaxing scented candles or incense, and update your bed linen to sound quality, non-synthetic sheets that will allow air to flow and your skin to breathe. You can also spritz your pillows with a sleep mist and ensure you have a comfortable mattress and pillows.

The idea is to create a cool, calming, and cozy atmosphere. Your room should be quiet, dark, and not too warm—around 70-72°F is the optimal room temperature for restful sleep. Open a window to allow fresh air to circulate—you can close it if it is noisy outside, but have it open for a while—and you may also want to get thicker or darker curtains to help block out light and noise.

Positive Sleep Practices

An adequate sleep schedule is vital to getting your recommended hours of sleep, and these science-based sleep hygiene practices will help you to create the best conditions for gaining a restful night's sleep. Some of these practices are done right before bed, others throughout the day—give them a go and see how your sleep cycle changes!

- Develop a consistent sleep schedule by going to bed and waking up at the same time every day (allow yourself half an hour or so of leeway). This is one of the most complex parts of sleep hygiene for many people, as some like to indulge in sleeping in at weekends, and others want to stay up late watching movies after a long day at work. However, it is crucial to create a sleep schedule and stick to it, as this will set your body's internal clock and sleep drive on a regular pattern, meaning your body will know when it can expect rest and prepare for it.

- Build your pre-bed routine. Fill the hour before you go to sleep with relaxing activities like meditation, reading, taking a warm bath, or listening to music. Avoid anything that overstimulates your mind and body. Meditation can be a great way to let the day's worries go so you can go to sleep with a clear mind.

- Turn the lights down low. Soft, dim lighting at night is far better than bright, harsh light that stimulates our minds and keeps the body from winding down. Start setting the bedtime mood after dinner by dimming the lights and lowering the brightness on electronics.

- Unplug from electronics at least 30 minutes before bed. Phones, laptops, and TVs stimulate our minds and disrupt our body clocks, which negatively impacts sleep. Also, you may pick up a worrying work email or see a social media post that causes you anxiety and gives you something to stew over all night when you should be sleeping. Don't risk it—put the phone on "Do not disturb" or block notifications and leave the worries for the next day.

- Exercise regularly—but not before bed! Try to get your exercise in earlier in the day so that when evening comes, your brain and body aren't stimulated anymore and could do with sleep to restore them.

- Avoid food and drink with caffeine or lots of sugar at least six hours before your bedtime— they can stay in the system for a long time and disrupt your sleep. If you want a hot beverage, have an herbal tea like chamomile or peppermint.

- Avoid sleep-disrupting foods too! Acidic, spicy, fatty, and fried foods, and heavy meals, can disrupt your digestion and make for an uncomfortable night's sleep. You may get indigestion and heartburn as your body struggles to break down food when it should be resting. Try not to eat heavily within five hours of going to bed.

- Cut down on alcohol before bed. Alcohol interferes with the sleep cycle, leading to restlessness and shallow sleep depth, so don't drink any within two hours of going to bed.

- Stay hydrated. Have a glass of water before going to bed —but not too much—as this will prevent dehydration overnight, so you'll wake up with more energy. It can also help cool your body, and if you have a cold or flu, a glass of hot water can relieve the symptoms, helping you get to sleep.

- Write a worry list. List things to do tomorrow or that are worrying you about the next day so they aren't on your mind when you're trying to sleep— they can wait!
- Use your bed for sleep and sex only. Avoid spending time in bed watching TV, eating, chatting, working, or social media scrolling—by keeping your bed for sleep and sex, you'll train your brain to see it as a place for rest and sleep only.
- Don't lie around waiting for sleep! If you haven't fallen asleep within 20 minutes of turning off the lights, get up and go to another room and engage in a relaxing activity like reading, a warm shower, or listening to music until you feel sleepy again. This stops you from getting frustrated by not sleeping and resets your body and mind.
- Skip the nap! If you have trouble falling asleep and staying asleep at night, avoid napping during the day, no matter how tired you feel. While a nap will boost your mood and energy in the short term, it will disrupt your body clock and make it harder to sleep at bedtime.

Start implementing these practices into your routine and lifestyle a few at a time, and see how your sleep changes! With time and effort, you'll feel stronger, healthier, and more energized and develop a more positive mindset around sleep. The two pillars of your life will feel supported and strong, and you'll have taken back control of the night and your body's essential natural cycle.

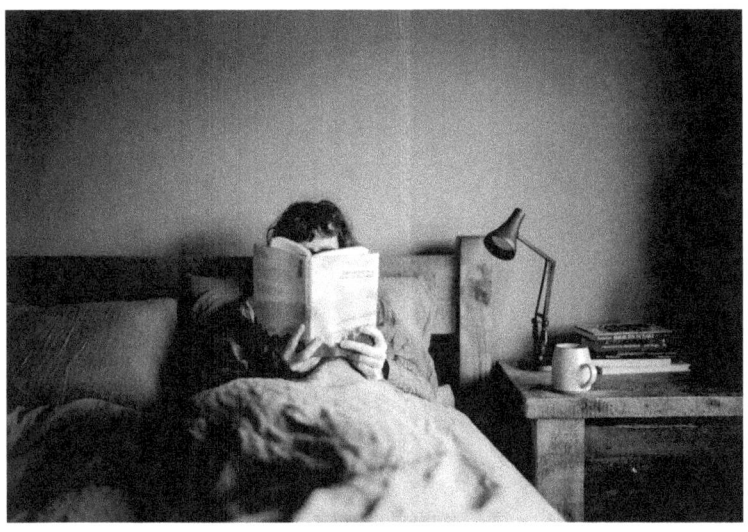

INTERACTIVE ELEMENT: SET YOUR SLEEP SCHEDULE

Let's start building your sleep schedule so you can begin your good sleep hygiene journey as soon as possible. Use this checklist in your Health Inventory to work your way through a nightly routine that promotes restful sleep and good bedtime habits.

- Have your final cup of caffeine six hours before bed.
- Have your dinner or final snack for the day at least four hours before bed.
- Dim the lights.
- Write your worry list—maybe with a soothing cup of chamomile.
- Open the bedroom window to let the fresh air in.
- Have a quick tidy-up in the bedroom.
- Have a warm bath or shower.
- Do your skincare routine and dress for bed with some calming music in the background.
- Set your alarm, turn off your phone—or at least the Wi-Fi—and unplug yourself from all electronics.
- Read, meditate, gently stretch, or listen to music or a soothing podcast until your bedtime.
- Drink a glass of water.
- Close the window if it is noisy or too cold.
- Get into bed and turn out the lights. Time to sleep!

The purpose of these good practices is to break the bad habits you may have gotten into that have been interfering with getting a good night's sleep. Bad habits creep up on us, and we often don't realize their negative impact until they are deeply ingrained in our routines. In the next chapter, we'll look at how to break them so you can retake control of your life.

5

SAYING "BYE" TO BAD HABITS

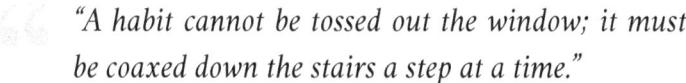
"A habit cannot be tossed out the window; it must be coaxed down the stairs a step at a time."

— MARK TWAIN

We've all got our bad habits, and try as we might to ignore them or justify them; let's face it, we know they're a problem! From little ones like endless social media scrolling to the big ones that cause emotional, physical, and mental issues for you and for others, they all need addressing if you're going to improve your life. Bad habits greatly impact our lives, wasting our time, money, and energy, interfering with productivity, encouraging toxic patterns, and preventing us from living up to our potential. A vital part of taking back control of your life is to break those bad habits once and for all. You'll need all your patience, willpower, and perseverance for this task, but you're not alone, and this chapter will guide you through understanding your bad habits, overcoming them, and building brilliant new ones.

DEFINING GOOD AND BAD HABITS

We have so many habits that we perform every single day that we don't even realize we have them. Habits are unconscious actions performed so many times that we do them effortlessly and without thinking, which is why we have such a problem identifying and breaking our bad habits. Since we aren't consciously controlling our actions but instead allowing our bodies to behave habitually, bad habits go unnoticed and unchecked. Bad habits can have detrimental effects on your physical, mental, and emotional health, including feelings of guilt, loss of sleep, heightened anxiety, poor eating patterns, and, in some cases, severe illness like cancer and heart disease.

Some bad habits are obvious, like smoking, drinking a lot of alcohol, or chewing your fingernails. In contrast, others are harder to identify because they form a small and routine part of our daily lives and can surely go unnoticed, but that doesn't make them worth ignoring. Some daily bad habits are far more noticeable for their impact on our lives, such as overspending, not exercising enough, and negative self-talk. These behaviors affect our bodies, minds, and budgets, and the short-term reward they give is not worth the long-term consequences of allowing them free rein over your life.

Some examples of everyday bad habits are:

- Poor money management, e.g., overspending, impulse buying, not saving
- Poor time management
- Not exercising
- Unhealthy eating
- Poor personal hygiene
- Slouching
- Scrolling endlessly on social media
- Checking your phone constantly
- Procrastinating
- Unhealthy sleep patterns
- Snacking every time you open the fridge
- Biting your nails
- Being late
- Lying
- People-pleasing
- Gossiping
- Staying in a toxic relationship or situation
- Overthinking

From this list, you might realize that sometimes a bad habit results from *inaction* or choosing *not* to do something that would be good for you, for example, exercising or eating healthily. Inaction is often the easiest option, requiring less commitment and effort than you might feel you can give at the moment. Because you're not actively choosing to indulge in a bad habit, you may not feel guilty or notice the negative impact of your behavior. Inaction is easier to explain away by making excuses such as being too tired or too busy, but these excuses are a sign that other bad habits are present in your life. As we'll see later in the chapter, actively working to change your bad habits is the only way to supercharge your life.

For all your bad habits, you're sure to have good ones too! Brushing your teeth properly, doing your skincare routine, and going to the gym are all good habits that you might already practice. Good habits, such as time management, healthy eating, and regular exercise, are the basis of a productive and positive routine that supports you in achieving your goals, keeping you healthy, boosting self-esteem, and reducing stress and anxiety. Good habits may take more effort to maintain, but the long-term results are incredible and life-changing.

Some examples of good habits to cultivate are:

- Good money management, e.g., budgeting, regularly saving
- Good time management
- Regular exercise
- Healthy eating
- Good personal hygiene
- Walking to the store rather than driving

- Maintaining a healthy sleep pattern
- Limiting TV and phone time
- Completing tasks in good time
- Being early
- Positive self-talk
- Self-reflection
- Saying "no"
- Removing yourself from toxic environments
- Giving people your full attention in conversation
- Setting boundaries

With good habits, the focus is on *action*. All the listed habits will take effort and perseverance, and you have to actively maintain and make time for them, but every single one positively affects your daily life.

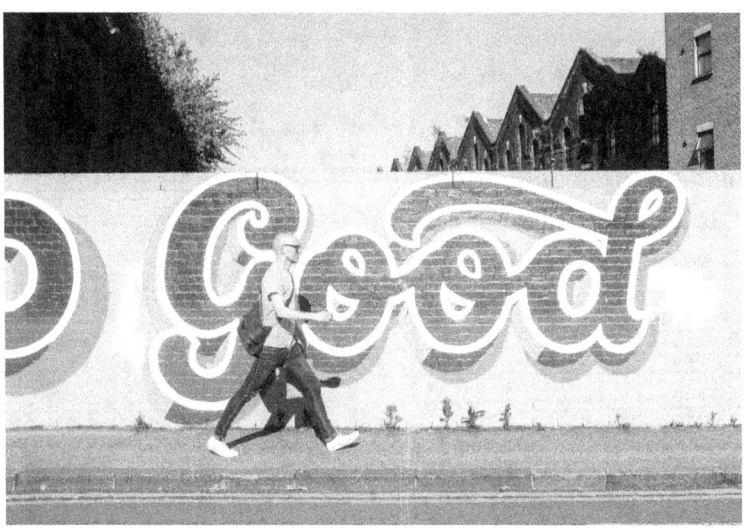

How Habits Are Formed

Bad habits form when the brain connects a **trigger**—like feeling anxious—with a **behavior**—having an alcoholic drink—and a **reward**—feeling more relaxed and less worried so you enjoy yourself more. Your brain quickly learns it can get short-term and immediate satisfaction from this behavior, and so it sends signals that cause you to repeat the action and behavior, chasing that feeling. Unfortunately, lousy habit behavior usually requires less energy and effort than good habit behavior, so bad habits often form far more effortlessly. There are other factors involved in creating bad habits too. Negative emotions, like those associated with certain mental disorders such as depression, can fuel bad habits, acting as cues for toxic and unhealthy behavior. Suppose you feel constantly depressed, anxious, or overwhelmed. In that case, you're more likely to pursue behaviors that bring immediate relief from these feelings rather than making positive life-style changes that require more energy and the rewards of which take longer to manifest, even though they would be more effective in helping you in the long term.

So, how do we break bad habits?

BREAKING BAD HABITS

Unsurprisingly, it is not half as easy to break bad habits as it is to form them, especially when they make us feel good or breaking them forces us to confront parts of our lives or ourselves that we would rather ignore. If you want to break bad habits, it's important not to feel ashamed or guilty about them but to approach them from a positive mindset that acknowledges them and why you need to change them. You have already improved your life from yesterday by choosing to break them today!

Breaking your bad habits will take commitment, perseverance, self-control, and self-reflection. That's a lot of energy and effort, so it's best to work on breaking only one or two bad habits at a time to avoid getting overwhelmed or burning out. It may seem as simple as just stopping doing something, but that can actually make you more likely to revert to your old behavior in a kind of withdrawal. Steadily working to remove the triggers and develop new routines to override the bad ones is far more effective and manageable.

Breaking Down Habit Breaking

Follow these steps for breaking bad habits:

1. **Identify your bad habit.** What behavior can you recognize is having a negative impact on your life?

Why do you want to change it? Understanding the effect it has on your life is an essential step to changing it. How will your life be better when you've broken the habit?

2. **Identify what triggers your bad habit.** Take a few days to track your bad habit and ask; when and where does it happen? Does it only occur in certain places or around certain people? Is it linked to another activity or event?

3. **Avoid or remove the trigger.** Change your behavioral pattern to remove the trigger and temptation. That might mean avoiding people, places, situations, or things that trigger you or simply not buying something, like cigarettes or sweets, anymore. Without the trigger, you will not activate the behavior.

4. **Replace the bad habit with a good one!** If it is hard to stop doing something, replacing it with something else—something better for you—can fill the gap, and in time, the urge to pursue the new habit will take over the old one.

There's a long road ahead of you, and along the way, there will be struggles, pitfalls, and setbacks that will threaten to derail your efforts, but try these tips for keeping on track to breaking that bad habit.

- **Start small and manageable.** Trying to break too many habits at once will be overwhelming, and you won't be able to give your full attention to them all. Instead, pick one or two that work together to break at a time.

- **Find ways to support yourself in your struggles.** It will be challenging at first, but you can help yourself by leaving reminders on sticky notes around the house, saying words of affirmation to yourself in the mirror, and putting up a list of the benefits of making the change so you can see it every day.

- **Find people to support you.** Family and friends can be beneficial as cheerleaders and goalkeepers for you. They can keep you on track to break your habit and may even want to join you in cracking the same habit for themselves! Some habits can seem impossible to break, but it is always a little easier with someone by your side.

- **Mentally prepare for setbacks and slip-ups.** Habits take a while to build up, so it makes sense they take even longer to break down, so don't expect it to happen overnight or without ups and downs. If you find yourself frustrated and falling back into old patterns, take a deep breath, identify where things went wrong, and see if there is a way to change your approach to breaking this bad habit that might be more effective. Most importantly, don't let doubt lead you to give up— remember that one bad day doesn't erase all your progress!

- **Reward your efforts and successes!** Keep yourself motivated to succeed with rewards and confidence boosts, and celebrate even small wins.
- **Don't be afraid to seek professional help.** Some bad habits, like addictions and compulsions, are tough to break on your own, and a mental health professional can be vital in overcoming them.
- **Change up your environment.** Walk a different route to avoid an expensive coffee shop, take the takeout menus down from the fridge, leave your journal on the coffee table, and avoid people and places that aren't supportive of you breaking your habit.
- **Filter out triggers.** Social media can be full of temptation and comparison, and it loves to show you things to distract you, so set filters to remove anything that might be a trigger or temptation from your feed.

There's no foolproof way to break a bad habit, but these tips should make the process easier and help keep you motivated and focused on your goal.

GROWING GOOD HABITS

Enough of the bad; now it's time for the good! When you replace bad habits with good ones, you open up your life to achieving your goals and potential. While bad habits make resisting temptation and negative behavior difficult, good habits flip that around and make resistance easier. It stops being a question of willpower and instead becomes a simple choice that requires no internal struggle—you just know what is right and what works best for you. Building healthy habits can seem like a mountainous and intimidating task—changing for the better constantly does—but breaking down the process into simple steps gives you more control and a more straightforward path.

1. **Set a specific goal for your good habit.** Be precise about what you'll do and when, and how often you'll do it. Doing a little towards your goal every day is a great way to make progress without overwhelming yourself.

2. **Plan the new habit into your routine with cues.** Cueing new behavior is a great way to make it a seamless part of your established routine, and it makes you less likely to forget to do it, for example, "Every day when I get home from work, I'll do twenty minutes of yoga in the living room before I make dinner." This is a firm and detailed plan and one that is more likely to stick and become a habit. The plan details the actions that will cue your behavior—in this case, returning home from work.

3. **Make it fun!** Find ways to make your new habit a fun and exciting part of your day; for instance, instead of just running on a treadmill—which can quickly grow dull even if it is effective—opt

instead for exercise that you enjoy and will look forward to doing, like a Zumba or Pilates class with a friend, or eat more fruit and vegetables by making flavor-packed smoothies.

4. **Be flexible.** In the early stages of changing habits, being strict can make the habit too difficult or rigid, so it doesn't fit into your lifestyle. Instead, have an ideal plan—like exercising every morning for half an hour—but be open to finding ways to fit it in elsewhere in your day. It might mean splitting it into two 15-minute sessions when you have time, but at least you'll do it! Being flexible makes it harder to throw off your plans, and it will keep you moving forward without frequent setbacks.

5. **Build a support network.** As with breaking bad habits, building good ones can be much easier with friends, family, and community to support your efforts, keep you motivated, and even join you on your quest. You could join a local running club, meal prep with your partner, or learn a language with a friend—there are so many options!

6. **Use reminders**, like Post-Its on the fridge or mirror or alarms and apps on your phone, to keep you focused on your good habit goal and to keep you from slipping back into bad habits. Your reminders could also be motivational, with

affirmations, commitments, or rewards written on them to help you maintain your efforts.

7. **Practice self-compassion.** Don't put too much pressure on yourself or engage in negative self-talk to shame yourself into action. Instead, stay focused on the positives of your habit journey, even when things are tough, and be gentle with yourself—remind yourself how far you've come and how hard you've worked, and tell yourself that you deserve the rewards you'll gain. Know that the only way to fail is to give up entirely and let setbacks fuel you to succeed.

Whatever your good habit goals are, there will be tough times, fun times, and with hard work and perseverance, success in the end. You already have everything you need to start today; willpower, intention, and self-belief. Harness your efforts and energy and pour them into making a better life for yourself! Think of habits as the ground beneath the two pillars of health. Bad habits make for uneven and unstable ground that cannot support the pillars of mental and physical health, so eventually, they fall, whereas good habits are robust and solid ground that keeps the pillars tall and supported, able to withstand the whirlwinds of life.

INTERACTIVE ELEMENT: BREAK A BAD HABIT!

For this final section of the chapter, let's create an action plan in your Health Inventory to break one of your bad habits and replace it with a good one. Starting small and working with the bad habit breakdown from earlier in the chapter, choose one bad habit that you know needs to change. For this example, let's try to stop using your phone before bed.

1. **Identify your bad habit.** Using your phone in bed before going to sleep.
2. **Identify what triggers your bad habit.** Perhaps it is boredom or feeling like you've missed out on something important happening in the world or your social group during the day.
3. **Avoid or remove the triggers.** Set app timers on all your social media apps to turn off an hour before bedtime. Turn your phone or the internet off before you start your bedtime routine. Put your phone on the other side of the room away from your bed. If you have a partner, ask them to do the same to help you with your goal.
4. **Replace the bad habit with a good one!** Have a book ready beside the bed and read for 30 minutes before turning off your light. Alternatively, you could listen to relaxing music or a guided bedtime meditation for 30 minutes.

Repeat this exercise for as many bad habits as you like, though try not to take on too much and overwhelm yourself with change. Start small, making little changes to your routine and behavior, and enjoy the big rewards of a life full of healthy habits! A favorite saying of ours that has become our mantra, small changes today make an immediate impact tomorrow!

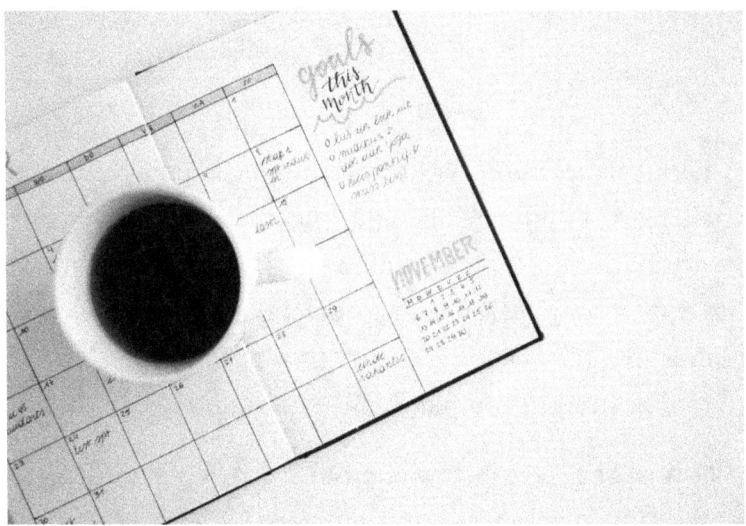

In the next chapter, we'll explore the power of self-awareness and its incredible impact on our mental and physical health.

SPREAD THE WORD: PHYSICAL AND MENTAL HEALTH GO HAND IN HAND – AND THEY CAN STRENGTHEN BOTH IN JUST 7 DAYS!

"True enjoyment is from the activity of the mind and exercise of the body; the two are ever united."

— WILHELM VON HUMBOLDT

Earlier in this book, we mentioned how quickly health challenges illuminate people on the inexorable link between their physical and mental health. They may develop a physical health problem, for instance, and realize that they lack the energy they need to socialize, go outdoors, or even complete daily tasks at home.

It also works the other way around. Anxiety and depression can be devastating, and someone experiencing these conditions can find it hard to maintain a job, stay active, or follow a healthy diet.

A myriad of studies have revealed that the link between the physical and mental cannot be ignored. For instance, one study published in *Nature Microbiology* reveals that there is a link between clinical depression and having low levels of specific gut bacteria. This is why so many experts recommend a fiber-rich diet—it can help you maintain good gut health!

Of course, working on your mental health by reducing stress, getting good sleep, and benefiting from the "feel-good hormones" released when you exercise, also improves your physical health.

Physical and mental health are two sides of the same coin. One cannot exist without the other. We are on a quest to ensure that everyone knows that they can make easy yet powerful changes that can revolutionize both. And we hope we can count on you to help us out.

We would appreciate it if you could leave a review of our book on Amazon, sharing your views on the mind-body connection.

Our hope is that someone who never makes time for themselves and tries to "soldier on" while neglecting their mind or body, understands two vital truths: they can make a change, and it is never too late to do so!

Give readers the motivation they need to develop a mindset that will inspire them to eat healthily, sleep well, and look forward to regular physical activity.

Scan the QR code for a quick review!

6

THE SELF-AWARE CHAMPION

"In our personal lives, if we do not develop our own self-awareness and become responsible for first creations, we empower other people and circum-stances to shape our lives by default."

— STEPHEN COVEY

W e spend so much of our time absorbed in other people's lives and actions, living in on-screen worlds and working on autopilot, and receiving vast amounts of information that we barely have time to process before we scroll further and find more. This busy and wirelessly connected existence makes it easy to lose awareness of our place in the world, our actions, their consequences, and how we feel about things. We become disconnected from what matters most—who we are and what we really need to live a happy, healthy life. Without self-awareness, we become passive and unfocused. We lose sight of our goals and ambitions. We can lose sight of our morals and ethics and instead find ourselves fitting into the patterns and needs of others at our own expense. Rebuilding and connecting with your self-awareness is a vital part of taking back control of your life and living it on your terms.

WHAT IS SELF-AWARENESS?

Self-awareness is making the conscious choice to evaluate your thoughts, needs, and feelings objectively so that you make focused and informed decisions and take action for your own well-being and others. It is knowing who you are as an individual, how you feel about things, what you want and need, and being aware of your power and place in this world. People who demonstrate good self-awareness are able to connect with their thoughts, emotions, and ethics and know when their behavior doesn't align with them and their own standards.

There are many benefits to improving your self-awareness. It is proven to help you build stronger relationships, be more creative and confident, make better decisions, and communicate more effectively with others. Self-aware people are less likely to lie and cheat and more likely to reap the rewards for their hard work by getting promotions (especially in leadership roles) and other jobs that offer them the chance to progress and use their skills to their full potential. Self-awareness gives you clarity about who you are, and this allows you to pursue your ambitions with focus, understanding, and self-belief. It is a powerful thing to be sure of yourself in a confused and overstimulated world. It gives you the strength to stand firm in your beliefs and goals and not be swayed into acting against your own interests by the opinions, fears, or influence of the world around you.

States of Self-Awareness

There are two states of self-awareness, one public and the other private. Cultivating strength in both states is crucial to taking ownership of yourself and your life.

Public

Public self-awareness relates to our awareness of how other people perceive us. You get a burst of public self-awareness when you are placed at the center of attention, for example, when giving a presentation in a meeting or at your wedding. In these situations, you may feel pressured to adhere to what you think society and the people around you expect of you. You may change your behavior to "fit in," acting against your own beliefs and personality —you might laugh at jokes you don't find funny or pretend to agree with something that offends you. Often, people will experience self-consciousness or evaluation anxiety—worrying about what others think of them—in these situations. Notwithstanding, if you have a strong sense of self-awareness, you'll be able to brush off these worries and feel confident being yourself or presenting your ideas and opinions, even if they don't "fit in."

Private

Do you know that feeling when your stomach lurches when you see your work crush or realize you forgot to send an important email or pay a bill? That is private self-awareness. Our internal self-awareness is how we perceive and understand our emotions, passions, values, and aspirations, adapt and fit into our environment, behave and react, and impact others. By reflecting on these areas, we build a sense of who we are, an authentic self:

- We can more effectively make decisions based on logic and good sense.
- We can regulate and channel our emotions proactively.
- We can maintain control and focus under pressure.

The danger of self-awareness is that it can become self-conscious when you start to doubt yourself and your worth. This leads you to hide your true self and instead present a "socially acceptable" persona that isn't a true reflection of who you are—in short, people never get to know the real you. This can be a way of protecting yourself, but it also significantly impacts your ability to take control of your life and find success in your relationships and ambitions.

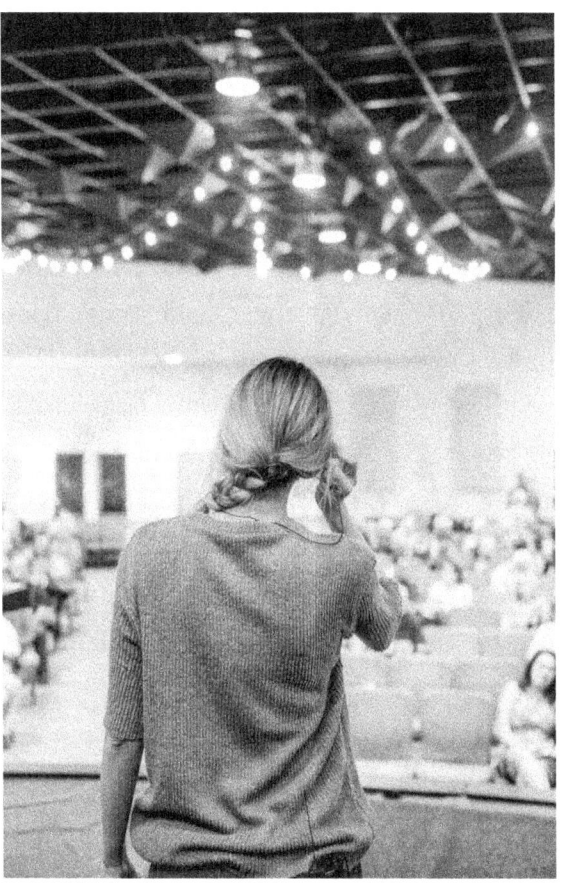

THE POWER OF SELF-AWARENESS ON THE PILLARS

Self-awareness can have a significant effect on our mental and physical health. With a healthy sense of self-awareness comes a healthy mind, which means a healthy body—everything is connected!

Mental

A lack of self-awareness can lead us to bottle up emotions. When those emotions are negative, it can lead to depression, anxiety, internalized anger, and resentment, which can then be turned outwardly as bullying or blaming others, leading to toxic relationships and loneliness or isolation. You could also end up people-pleasing at your own expense. Also, excessive self-consciousness can lead to social anxiety disorder, which can be debilitating. This shows how important it is to work to improve your self-awareness to benefit your mental health. Some of the significant benefits of a good sense of self-awareness are:

- Improved communication, which means you can express yourself and your needs more clearly.
- Builds empathy and understanding, promoting positive relationships.
- Improved self-confidence so we feel happier in ourselves and our appearance.

- Decreased stress since you are more assured of your ability to cope under pressure.
- Improved emotional intelligence (EQ): The ability to regulate your emotions so they don't rule you and express them in a healthy and productive way.

With private self-awareness and a healthy sense of self, you are more likely to have job and relationship satisfaction and a sense of control over your social, professional, and personal life, which leads to a happier and more stable mindset and a low likelihood of developing depression or anxiety.

Physical

The physical benefits of self-awareness on the body are directly linked to the mental benefits. Self-aware people work to improve themselves, which means they look after their bodies better, exercise regularly, participate in active pursuits, and find it easier to maintain healthy eating habits. The grand connection between gut health and mental health means that self-awareness can improve symptoms of IBS and aid digestion. The positive lifestyle that comes with good self-awareness comes with happiness, which floods your body with happy hormones that give you more energy and curb your cravings—and let's face it, happy, confident people just look better!

HOW TO DEVELOP YOUR SELF-AWARENESS

Developing self-awareness means opening yourself up to experiences, people, emotions, and reflections that encourage you to assess yourself and your actions. It can be very eye-opening and sometimes scary, but the point is to grow and improve, to understand yourself better. Here are some ways you can develop your self-awareness every day:

- Journaling is extremely helpful! Noting down what triggers positive feelings for you will help you pursue good people and experiences. Journaling also helps you to evaluate your feelings, process emotions and experiences, and be more mindful.
- Meditation is excellent for centering and focusing the mind so that you can dig deep into a feeling, problem, or thought within yourself, rather than being distracted by the external world. It can guide you to deeper understanding and new perspectives and help you to listen to your inner voice so you can form your own ideas. With meditation, you can also take the time to be present with just yourself and your emotions, without judgment or pressure.
- Ask for feedback and work to improve based on it. On a personal level, you could ask other people how they see you or ask a coworker or manager to

give you feedback on your performance. You may not like what you hear, but accepting feedback and working on it will help you develop understanding and awareness.

- Check in with yourself. Take a moment to pause and check in on where you are and what you are feeling. You can do this anytime, but it is advantageous in times of stress, panic, and high emotion.
- Be curious! Explore and experience as much as possible to develop opinions, skills, and confidence.
- Open yourself up and drop your defenses. Allow things to affect you, and don't avoid something on the chance you may get hurt.
- Keep learning! Building skills and discovering interests will reveal new things about you.
- Try to see things from other people's perspectives. When you are upset or angry with someone, remember they don't see things the way you do and are in a different situation. Approach them with empathy, ask them to explain their point of view, and be willing to hear their feedback and side of things.
- Look at your life and ask yourself, what am I learning and doing that serves me? What do I need, or need to do, to obtain what I want? Pursue the answer!

Self-awareness ensures you go through life with your eyes and mind open and with the confidence to be yourself everywhere you go. Self-awareness will equip you to tackle problems with understanding rather than emotion, and you'll be able to set and pursue your goals with clarity and purpose—something that we'll explore in the next chapter. Self-awareness is a solid core for the two pillars, a hidden support that keeps them and you standing firm against damaging external forces that try to keep you from reaching your full potential and harnessing control of your life.

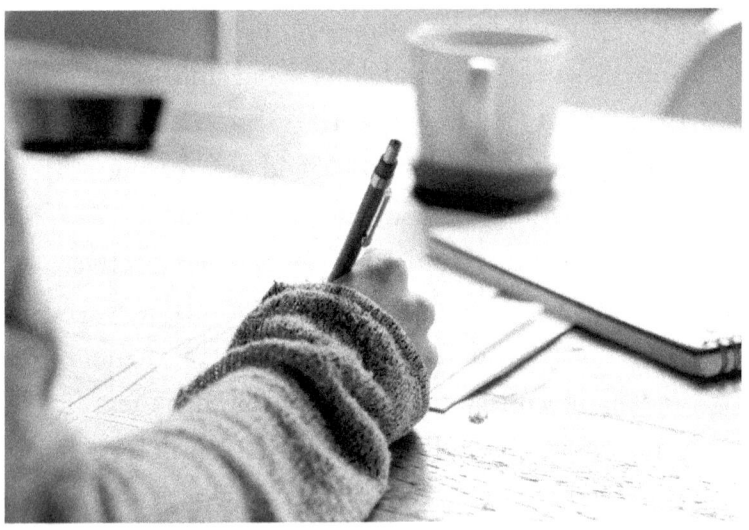

INTERACTIVE ELEMENT: THE SELF-AWARENESS WORKSHEET

Find a quiet and comfortable place to sit where you can focus. Grab your Interactive Health Inventory, a pen, and a cup of soothing tea. You will be working your way through a series of questions designed to enhance your self-awareness and encourage reflection. Answer honestly, taking your time to listen to your feelings and understand your desires. Allow this worksheet to take you on a tour of yourself and your life without judgment. Are you ready?

Breathe in... breath out...

Personality

1. What do you consider to be your best and worst traits/qualities?
2. What qualities do you wish you had?
3. What do you consider to be your five greatest strengths and weaknesses?
4. What do you like most about yourself?
5. What is one thing that you would change about yourself?
6. What song represents you?
7. What fictional character do you most identify with?

Values

8. What are the ten things that are most important to you?
9. How much time and energy do you devote to these things?
10. What do you believe is your most outstanding achievement?
11. What do you look for in a friend?
12. What are five things you like and five you dislike?
13. Who do you most admire in real life?
14. What fictional characters do you most admire?
15. What do you think someone would admire in you?
16. What do you fear?

Life and Goals

17. What is your idea of happiness?
18. What are three of your life goals?
19. What is a dream you have always had?
20. What is keeping you from achieving your dreams and goals?
21. What are you most proud of?
22. What talent would you most like to have?
23. Where would you love to visit?
24. What activities bring you the most joy?
25. What is your biggest regret?

Relationships

26. What is your idea of the perfect relationship with a friend, a romantic partner, and a family member?
27. Who can you be yourself around?
28. What has been the best moment of any relationship you have had? It doesn't have to be romantic!
29. What has been the most challenging moment?
30. What do you need most from a partner?
31. What do you offer a partner?

Appearance and Health

32. Do you respect your body and care for it?
33. What are your best physical attributes?
34. What outfit or item of clothing makes you feel happiest/best?
35. What is one area of your health you could improve?
36. When were/are you most content in your body?

Public

37. Do you always put others' needs ahead of your own?
38. Do you need approval from others?
39. What do you think people like most and least about you?
40. When you have done something wrong, do you ignore it and hope it goes away or try to fix it?
41. Do you avoid confrontation or speak up for yourself?

Based on your answers and reflections, identify areas you think self-awareness could improve your life, career, relationships, and health.

One final task. Can you remember a recent time when you lacked self-awareness? What impact did it have on you and others? How can you change your behavior and communication for next time? What can you do differently?

It's time to look outside of yourself now, at the world and life you have created, and decide if you're on the path to achieving your goals and dreams. In the next chapter, you'll learn how to set goals effectively and realistically to take control of your future.

7

MOVING THE GOAL POST

"It is good to have an end to journey toward; but it is the journey that matters, in the end."

— URSULA K. LE GUIN, *THE LEFT HAND OF DARKNESS*

Goals are an essential part of life. They give us purpose and direction, help us achieve significant milestones in our lives and careers, and give us a sense of fulfillment, achievement, and progress. With goals, we can gain sight of what we want and need in life, leading us to save resources and energy on less pivotal pursuits. We can strive for big goals that shape our lives, like buying a house, getting a promotion, or having a child. Yet just as vital, we must have small everyday goals that are stepping stones to those larger goals, like saving money and eating healthily.

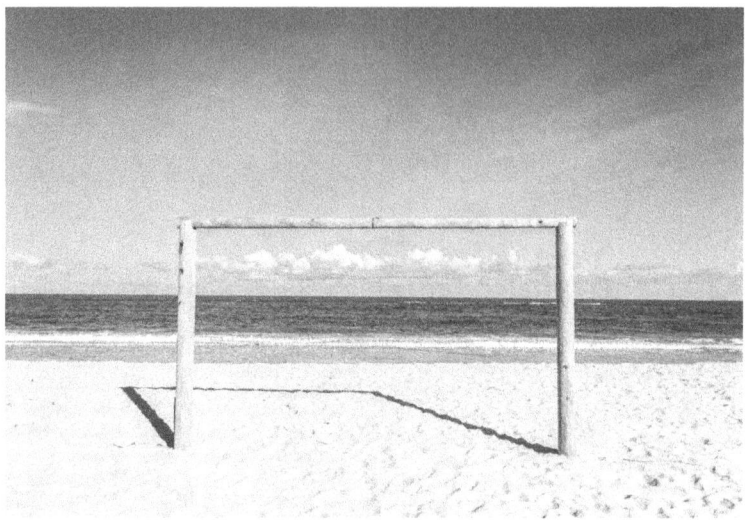

GOAL POWER

Goals are the destination at the end of the road, the roadmap of our lives. Sometimes the road is straight and easy, but more often, the road is full of hazards—hills to climb, cliffs to fall from, crossroads, and unexpected detours. Without goals, we would drift through life without purpose or direction, staying in places or situations that hold us back or hurt us, never taking risks or reaching for our desires. Our goals help us to prioritize our actions and understand what we value most in life, and they hold us accountable, even if we fail, forcing us to reflect on our actions and wants. They also help us to focus our efforts so that we don't waste our time, money, and energy on unimportant and unproductive ventures. Above all, they keep us motivated in the face of the many challenges of life, challenges that threaten to derail our goals and shuffle our priorities.

Goal Categories

You're probably juggling any number of goals in any number of areas all the time, and this is a good thing. It means you are aware of needing change in many areas of your life and are not limiting your progress. Juggling multiple goals can be overwhelming, so let's break it down and start by looking at the seven main categories of life goals:

1. **Health goals:** Losing weight, getting fit, going to the gym, and beating an illness are all common health goals.
2. **Professional goals:** These might include getting a promotion, changing careers, finding your dream job, and even leaving a toxic one.
3. **Educational goals:** You spend your whole life learning, so these goals don't stop with graduation! In adult life, they could be learning a new skill, seeking out knowledge on an area of interest, or taking a course at work.
4. **Financial goals:** In an expensive world, it is important to set financial goals, including saving money, budgeting, and paying off debts.

5. **Relationship goals:** Setting goals for your relationships is crucial to keeping them strong, healthy, and fulfilling for everyone.

6. **Personal growth goals:** These goals are aimed at becoming the best version of yourself, at making you feel good. They include making more time for things you enjoy or developing your personal style and appearance.

7. **Spiritual goals:** Goals for strengthening the spirit and bringing happiness into your life, such as volunteering, meditating, and practicing mindfulness.

It is usual to have long- and short-term goals in each of these areas simultaneously. Some may take priority or be more urgent than others, while some may require years of work to attain. Achieving goals in all areas is vital to living a healthy and fulfilling life and taking control of your life.

SETTING SMART GOALS

Whether your goals are short- or long-term, careful planning and clear goal-setting is the key to achieving them. SMART goals are a way of setting goals to make them as achievable and realistic as possible—they help give you clarity about your aims, keep your goals aligned with your values, and ensure your goals fit with your lifestyle and resources. So, what makes SMART goals smart?

SMART goals must be:

- **S**pecific
- **M**easurable
- **A**chievable
- **R**elevant
- **T**ime-bound

Specific

In order to make achievable goals, you need to make them specific. Making them specific helps avoid wasting time or effort on things that don't actually help you towards your goal. It breaks the goal down, making it more precise and less intimidating. It can also help you understand why the goal is paramount to you in the first place.

Answer these six questions to help make your goal specific:

1. **Who** is involved in achieving the goal/plan?
2. **What** goal do you want to achieve?
3. **Where** will your goal be pursued and completed?
4. **When** will you start the plan, and **when** will you attain the goal?
5. **Which** obstacles may hinder your progress and success?
6. **Why** do you want to accomplish this goal?

Measurable

By making your goals and progress measurable, SMART goals hold you accountable, help you track and define your progress, and keep you to your deadlines. Being able to measure your progress will keep you motivated, as even if you have a bad month, you'll still be able to see how far you've come in the months before.

Achievable

For your goal to be successful, it needs to be realistic, taking into consideration your skills and abilities, your resources, and any factors that could hinder you from achieving your goal. Your goal should offer the chance to challenge or develop your skills so you can progress towards it, but don't take on anything you don't have the time or resources for—this will only make achieving your goal harder!

Relevant

Keep your goals relevant to your lifestyle, ambitions, and needs, and stay in control of them. You might need support from other people at various stages, but keeping things in your hands as much as possible means you retain ownership of your success. When setting your goal, use these questions to make sure it is relevant:

- Does pursuing this goal seem worth the time and effort needed?
- Is now the right time to be pursuing this goal? Do you have other commitments or goals that take priority?
- Are you the right person to achieve this goal?
- Are you in a position to achieve it?

Time-bound

Setting a target date for achieving your goal makes you substantially more likely to achieve it! Deadlines keep you focused and accountable for how you use the time leading up to them, and you're less likely to procrastinate if you have a strict time frame. Have a realistic target date, but also consider what you can do in six months, six weeks, or even what you can do today to get one step closer to your goal. If your goal is long-term, think about giving yourself time to accomplish the short-term goals that contribute to it.

SMART TIP! Be careful not to set goals that rely on other people's efforts or that someone else has power over, for example, getting hired for your dream job. Ultimately, getting hired is up to the recruiter, not you, but your goal can be "Build the skills and experience I need to be a perfect candidate for the role," which *is* something you do have control over.

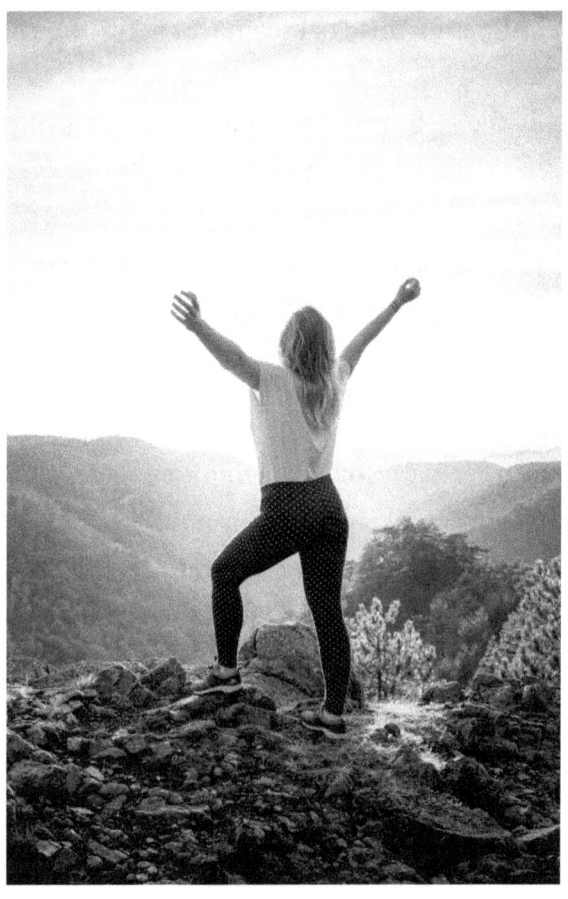

The Benefits of SMART Goals

SMART goals are a very effective tool for many reasons. They keep you motivated by setting a realistic and achievable time frame to work towards that allows for your lifestyle and any setbacks that might occur. This time frame also inspires action. Since you can't keep putting your goal off and waiting for "the right moment," you must get started and see it through. SMART goals also help to keep the end goal in focus throughout the journey, serving as a reminder that the hard work will be worth it in the end. The specificity of SMART goals helps you to plan the best way to achieve your goal in advance, making the journey to success as straightforward and achievable as possible. They encourage you to prioritize your goals and efforts, and they can help you identify why you may be struggling to achieve goals. They also can help you find ways to improve driving you towards success. SMART goals also force you to push the limits of your comfort zone by ensuring there's no room for excuses! By being time-bound, there's no room for procrastination and the comfort zone of putting off things you are worried about. Plus, you're more likely to achieve more of your goals and use your time wisely with the finish line in sight and getting closer every day!

Sadly, even with all these benefits and the higher chance of success, life's unexpected and unavoidable events can occur, and failure can still happen—so how do we deal with it and use it to fuel our efforts rather than ruin them?

MY GOAL FAILED... NOW WHAT?

For many people, the fear of failing is the main reason they don't set clear goals—it is easier to make excuses for failure if there is no plan to follow or deadline to meet—but failure is, unfortunately, a standard part of adult life. You'll never progress or achieve anything if you try to avoid it. Living with, and growing from, your failures is an essential skill to cultivate if you desire to live a happy and fulfilled life.

There are many reasons for failing to achieve a goal. Sometimes you work hard but don't quite get there, the universe seems to work against you, and the chances you were counting on don't materialize, you misjudge what you are able to give to the goal effort and fall short, or someone else gets there first. Everyone fails at some point, but the ones who will succeed are the ones who don't wallow in their misery and failure. Instead, they use it to fuel their energy to regroup, reassess, reflect, and move on positively and productively. Let's explore some ways you can use failure as a stepping-stone to success next time:

- Perform a post-mortem on your failure. Failure has signaled that there was something wrong with your goal, plan, or efforts, and if you ignore these signals, you'll only keep making the same mistakes. Doing a post-mortem is asking yourself, "Why did I fail?" and searching for understanding. It might be you overestimated your abilities or didn't work hard enough, you procrastinated too much, or you didn't give yourself enough time— don't place blame. Just identify and acknowledge where you went off track. Understanding why you fail will help you avoid those mistakes next time.

- Take a break and get away. If you feel too disheartened and anxious to try again immediately, give yourself space and time away from your goal before trying again. Taking a step back will help you see it with fresh eyes and give your brain time to refocus and work through the problem independently. Make sure you come back, though. Don't abandon your goal!
- Ask yourself the hard questions. Brutal honesty will help you identify where you went wrong, so ask yourself:

  o "Has what I've done justified this outcome?"
  o "Is this how people who have been successful in this area have done it?"
  o "If I continue doing things the way I am, will I achieve my goal?"

Use the answers to change your efforts and strategy to go after what you want!

- Seek feedback from someone successful in achieving this or a similar goal! How did they do it, and how did they overcome their problems pursuing it? Ask for advice, and act on it.
- Reflect on your progress and the positives instead of focusing solely on the negatives of failure. See how far you came towards achieving your goal,

and remember that experience and effort are success too.

- Reevaluate your motivations. Maybe you failed because you lost your steam or the goal needed to realign with changes in your life or needs. Check-in with yourself and assess whether the goal is still what you want to pursue or if it needs to change a bit to reflect new experiences, knowledge, or other factors.
- Be kind to yourself. Self-empathy—not self-pity—will help you to avoid blame and negative thoughts that can lead to you abandoning your goal entirely. Remember, you're only human, and so is every successful person to do it before you—if they can do it, so can you!

Your goals shape your life and future, guiding you through difficult times and leading you toward the light of success. The two pillars of your life, mental and physical health, are instrumental in pursuing your goals. Improving and maintaining good mental health will give you the strength and clarity to know what you want and focus on your goals. It will enable you to solidify your self-belief, to know that you deserve to achieve your goals as much as anybody else. Looking after your physical health will give you a strong, energized body that can take you on your adventures and bear the weight and challenges of your endeavors. Taking control of your life means letting your failures inform your actions in a positive way that keeps you moving forward toward your dreams and desires, leading you to the life you've always wanted.

INTERACTIVE ELEMENT: SET A SMART GOAL!

Let's start taking control right now! Based on your goals from chapter one, choose something to develop into a SMART goal, one step at a time. We'll use the goal of getting promoted at work as an example. Grab a pen and your Interactive Health Inventory and take your time to work through each step of the SMART process.

1. Make your goal **SPECIFIC**:

   a. Who is involved in achieving the goal/plan? E.g., me and my superiors who will interview me.
   b. What goal do you want to achieve? E.g., be promoted to head of the department.
   c. Where will your goal be pursued and completed? E.g., My workplace.
   d. When will you start the plan, and when will you achieve the goal? E.g., I will start now by taking courses to increase my skillset, then apply for promotion in two years.
   e. Which obstacles may hinder your progress and success? E.g., How much of my spare time I can give to taking courses to advance my skills and experience and whether I interview well.

f. Why do you want to achieve this goal? E.g., I want to advance in my career, lead the team, and enjoy the pay rise!

With these answers in mind, write your goal clearly: "I will develop the skills and experience to demonstrate my ability to be the head of the department in my organization."

1. How will you **MEASURE** your goal? What will be the milestones that show you are making progress? For example: "Complete the necessary courses for the promotion and ask for performance feedback from a supervisor."
2. How can you make your goal **ACHIEVABLE**? What skills, abilities, and resources do you have or need to achieve your goal? What may hinder your progress that you can prepare for now? For example: "I will need to complete a course in… and… in order to meet the promotion requirements. I need to spend an hour every day studying the course materials."
3. Is your goal **RELEVANT** to your life right now?
4. Give yourself **TIME**. You need a clear and reasonable time frame for success. For example: "I will apply for promotion in two years and complete one course every six months."

This process can take time and research but work through each stage carefully to ensure you are building an achievable and motivating plan for your goal. When you've done one, try doing another!

Setting your goals is a great start, but you need to make room for them in your daily life to progress toward them. One way to make room for attaining your goals and removing unnecessary anxiety from your life, is decluttering and clearing out chaos in your home. Keeping a healthy and clean home is vital to maintaining control and direction in life, and in the next chapter, we'll discuss putting together an action plan to clean and declutter your home.

8

KEEPING A HEALTHY HOME

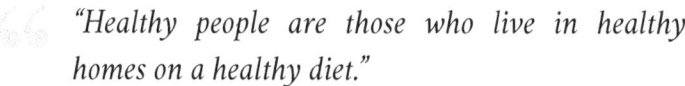 *"Healthy people are those who live in healthy homes on a healthy diet."*

— IVAN ILLICH

Your home is your haven. It is your safe place where you can relax, unwind, and enjoy entertaining friends and family. You should be able to come home from work to a clean, tidy, tranquil, and welcoming home that helps ease the day's burdens. It should inspire peace and positivity, but it is easy to let negativity in, and once it is in, it can be hard to get it out. When this happens, the home becomes just another realm of anxiety and unproductivity, and a cycle of toxic home habits quickly begins as the clutter takes over and the effort to clean and tidy becomes increasingly overwhelming and impossible. This chapter will help you reclaim your home and make it a sanctuary for your mind and body.

YOUR HOME AND YOUR HEALTH

When your mental and physical health is anguishing, your home inevitably does as well, becoming messier and more cluttered as you add to the pile of clothes on the chair, dirty dishes in the sink, or papers on the coffee table. When you're physically and mentally exhausted, and as anxieties, illnesses, and obligations increase, your energy levels decrease, and you add onto the piles until your home is full of seemingly unconquerable mountains of clutter. At this point, throwing in the towel and letting your house be taken over is effortless, but that is the *worst* thing you can do for your health. There are many benefits for the mind and body in taking back control of your home, so let's explore them and get motivated!

Benefits for the Body

While the outside world may seem treacherous and unclean, your home can be just as unsafe, and since you spend such a large part of every day in your home, you can undoubtedly put your health in danger if you do not keep it clean. A dirty home encourages pests, mold, dust, and allergies, which all cause health problems. Bacteria spread rapidly in a dirty environment, and pests carry viruses, so offering them the perfect habitat to explore and make their home is a surefire way to get sick. Regularly wiping down surfaces, door handles, and food preparation and storage areas can make your home far safer in just a few minutes.

An unclean kitchen is hazardous. Bacteria and flies will riot if you leave dirty dishes, soiled tea towels, and basins full of used water lying around. You're also more prone to food poisoning from cross contamination and bacteria if your appliances, fridge, and cooking utensils aren't kept clean. Mold and dampness can cause lung problems if left untreated, so it's best to deal with them as soon as you spot them. Keep your home airy and uncluttered to stop mold and dampness from growing, spreading, and hiding.

On a slightly slapstick note, a cluttered house is a mine-field of things to trip over! You can hurt yourself easily by slipping on a greasy or wet floor or by tripping over a mess and clutter left lying around. Save yourself the bumps, bruises, and even breaks, by keeping the floors clean and clear of debris and wiping up any spills as soon as you make them.

Cleaning is also a great form of exercise. You can really work up a sweat doing a deep clean or even just a vacuum, and if you put music on and dance while you do it, it's even more fun and effective! If you're unable to leave the house or exercise at home, cleaning is a superb way to get your blood moving and your muscles working.

Studies have shown that you sleep better in a decluttered room too. You can relax and unwind much more effectively in a room where you aren't looking at piles of unfolded laundry or an errant sock that you know you should pick up but you just got comfy. A tidy room also allows clean air to circulate better, and clean bedding will keep bed bugs and other pests away. Better sleep makes for a healthier and more energized body!

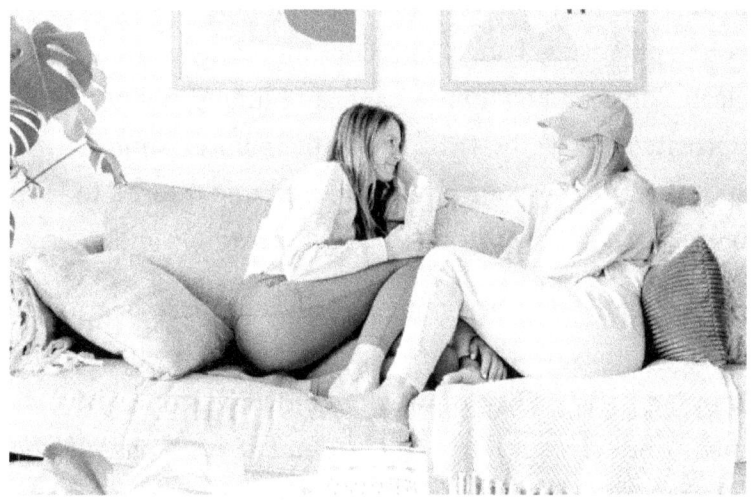

Benefits for the Mind

Your environment has a significant impact on your mind. Stressful, high-pressure environments make you stressed and anxious, while tranquil settings make you feel relaxed and safe—your home should be the latter. Keeping your home clean and tidy makes it a less stressful and more calming environment, and one you won't feel like you have to spend hours cleaning on the weekend when you'd rather be doing anything else. Also, a tidy house will save you time looking for things because everything will be where it should be.

A messy home or workplace can considerably impact concentration, creating mental clutter to match the physical. It draws your focus and distracts your attention, which can cause you to procrastinate and forget things. Keeping your home clear of clutter will help you concentrate and make doing the chores easier since you won't have to keep picking up and moving things to clean underneath them. Tidiness also helps to avoid overstimulation. You already have so much drawing your attention —phones, computers, TVs, social media—that it's nice to have a space clear of distractions and stimulations that you can decompress and focus on yourself in.

Putting care and attention into your surroundings is a form of self-care and self-love—you are showing yourself that you *deserve* peace and gifting yourself health and happiness at home. The mood-boosting energy of a tidy home is fantastic, not to mention decluttering and cleaning gives you a sense of achievement, so even on an adverse or unproductive day, you can feel you have accomplished something just by tidying a room. This feeling of accomplishment boosts happiness and self-image. Maintaining a healthy home also allows you a sense of control over at least one area of your life. Feeling powerless and unfocused is terrible for mental health, but exerting your will by managing your home can be a great way to feel capable, productive, and in control.

It might seem strange, but cleaning and tidying can be a very efficient form of meditation, especially for anyone who finds it challenging to sit and self-reflect in silence for a long time. Instead, you can keep your hands busy clearing the physical clutter and allow your brain to take a needed break from the mental chaos, giving you precious time and headspace to escape your anxieties and be present in the moment.

Finally, you're more likely to invite people into your home to socialize if your home is welcoming and clean, so you'll be able to spend more time with your friends and avoid the stress of a last-minute, frantic tidy-up when someone announces they are dropping by. Feelings of isolation and loneliness are damaging to mental health and often increased by a sense of shame or guilt about the appearance of your home, but keeping on top of your cleaning routine will free you up to opening your doors to the world and strengthening your relationships.

MAKE YOUR HOME A SANCTUARY

Refreshing your home and banishing the mess and clutter may seem an overwhelming task, especially if it has been a while since you tried or you just haven't had the time or energy, so let's break down the process into smaller steps to take back your space and make your home a peaceful paradise again.

Declutter

The first step to finding sanctuary is to eliminate the clutter and chaos that is filling the space with negative energy and making the task seem impossible. Decluttering is more than just tidying up—it is about removing objects and debris that cause anxiety and bring no joy to your home. Often clutter takes the form of hoarded possessions like clothes, electronics, and decorations, which get tossed about and overload the cabinets and surfaces so you can't find the stuff you need or want. Decluttering your house will show you the things that matter, make your life better, help you to bring order to your home, and improve the quality of your life. Here are some tips for decluttering to make it a straightforward and productive process:

- Before you start, ensure you have plenty of boxes and trash bags ready. As you declutter, segregate things to keep and donate into separate boxes. Only throw away broken items or anything too dirty to save.
- Pick **one** area of the house to start in, not a whole room, just a corner or a cabinet. Starting small makes the task less intimidating and helps to focus your efforts and avoid distractions. You can work

your way around the room and the house, area by area, for as long as you like—it could take one day or over a week. Just be sure to go at your own pace.

- Sort through objects individually, deciding whether to keep, donate, or throw them away. Only keep things that make you feel happy, are essential or valuable, and are used often.
- Have a microfiber cloth or cleaning wipes handy to wipe down surfaces and objects as you go.
- Donate unwanted items as soon as possible so they aren't hanging around the house.
- Use baskets, boxes, and wire zipties to make everything neat and keep surfaces clear.
- If you can't decide whether to keep or donate something, give yourself a deadline to use it, for example, three months. Let it go if you haven't used, worn, or needed it at the end of the three months.

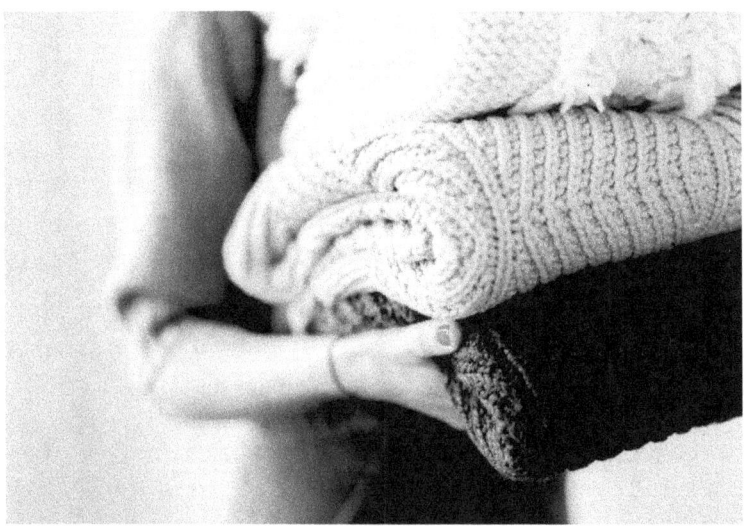

Conquer the Cleaning

It is easy to feel defeated, unmotivated, and overwhelmed in the face of such an arduous task as cleaning the house, so use these cleaning tips and tricks to take back control of your home's health and defeat the dirt.

- Set a timer for a realistic amount of time to clean —enough time that you can make progress but won't get overwhelmed. Get as much done as you can in that time. Even just ten minutes of cleaning one room a day can make a huge difference, and that ten minutes is effortless to slip into your daily routine, and it will fly by before you know it.
- Pick one area, or object to clean, and focus your energy on that. Sorting the laundry is a great example. Appliances like the refrigerator, oven,

and shower take more effort to clean than anything else, so make sure to give yourself plenty of time with them.

- Give each room a day of the week for its turn to be cleaned—this way, you'll be able to keep the rooms on a constant cleaning rotation that should keep dirt and mess from building up throughout the house.
- Use eco friendly plant based cleaning sprays, wipes, and microfiber cloths to make cleaning easier.
- Put on an energizing playlist as loud as you like to keep your spirits and energy up while you clean!
- Prioritize the cleaning tasks that have a positive and noticeable effect on the space, for example, changing your bed sheets or cleaning the oven. They will show you the rewards of your efforts and motivate you to keep going!
- Ask for help! Having someone to work through chores with you makes it more fun and the task more manageable.
- Make a thorough list of what to clean in every room and work your way through it—checking off your cleaning accomplishments will feel more rewarding and productive!

Decor and Design

How you decorate your home has an incredible and often overlooked impact on your health. There are lots of ways to improve your physical and, especially, your mental health with simple design and decor choices, such as:

- Fill up empty space with houseplants! They not only give out needed oxygen that improves air quality and aids concentration, but they are a fun project, and keeping them healthy and alive is very rewarding. Like humans, plants need love and care, so share a little with them, and they'll give it back.
- Use light and cool colors to energize and enlarge a room or warm and dark colors for cozy spaces.
- Don't rely on ceiling lights, which can be harsh and overstimulating, especially in the evening. Use lamps or fairy lights as night draws in, and candles can be very calming too—only don't forget to blow them out before bed!
- Fill your home with soothing scents! Scents like vanilla, lavender, rose, and cinnamon are remarkably calming and will make your home feel fresh and welcoming. Sage smudging is a great way to remove negative energy from your home too!

- Decorate to encourage joy! Bright colors and lively wall art can boost mood and energize your home.
- Choose blankets, duvet covers, and pillowcases in soft, breathable fabrics like cotton or linen to encourage cool and comfortable sleep.
- Keep to an aesthetic when decorating and choosing furniture. This will give your home a cohesive and controlled atmosphere which will help you focus and be more motivated to keep it tidy.
- Give yourself *space* to move and think. Encourage air and energy flow around the home, and don't fill the space with objects and furniture. Moving around should be easy, and less stuff means less to clean!

You don't need the stress of making considerable changes to your decor all at once, and you certainly don't need to rack up the cost of replacing all the furniture—take your time, work with what you've got, and add to your home at your own pace and within your budget.

INTERACTIVE ELEMENT: YOUR ROOM-BY-ROOM DEEP CLEAN CHECKLIST

Deep cleaning is an essential—and rewarding—task for maintaining a healthy home, but it can be intimidating and time-consuming at the same time. Luckily, staying on top of your weekly cleaning routine makes deep cleaning more manageable and less overwhelming. A deep clean aims to focus your energy on eliminating the dirt, dust, and grime that can get overlooked in your everyday cleaning efforts. You'll be cleaning the hard-to-reach areas that are typically missed quite easily and dusting and scrubbing the house from top to bottom. While some rooms, like the bathroom and kitchen, need a thorough wiping down every week, you'll only need to perform a deep clean on the whole house once or twice a year.

You will need:

- A mop and bucket
- Cleaning cloths—microfiber cloths are great!
- Multipurpose cleaner
- Rubber gloves
- A vacuum cleaner
- Toothbrush—for corners and drains, etc.
- Telescopic duster
- White vinegar
- Baking soda
- Window and glass cleaner

- Non-scratch scrubbing pads

Use the following checklist and the supplies above to deep clean every room in your home thoroughly, one at a time. You can break it down and do one room a month to make deep cleaning more manageable.

Bedroom

- Launder all the bedding, including the blanket/duvet and pillows, and wipe down the bed frame.
- Refresh your mattress. Sprinkle it all over with baking soda, leave it for an hour, then vacuum it thoroughly—this will eliminate odors. Don't forget to flip the mattress and do the other side!
- Declutter your closets and drawers, dust and wipe inside, and leave them open to breathe and dry well while you sort through your clothes.
- Dust, vacuum, and wipe down the baseboards and windowsills.
- Vacuum the curtains or blinds and clean the windows.

Kitchen

- Empty out your cabinets, and pantry shelves, and thoroughly wipe them down inside and all over the doors. While they dry and air out, go through the contents, throw away anything out of date, and wipe any residue off bottles and containers.
- Clear your counters of appliances, clean and dry them and the backsplash. Wipe down the appliances, and only put back what you use daily —find homes in cabinets and out of sight for everything you use less often.
- Deep clean your large appliances—fridge, freezer, stove, oven, and dishwasher—inside and out (you may need special cleaning supplies for the oven and dishwasher.) Pull them away from the wall to clean behind and beneath them if you can.
- Scrub and wipe down the sink.
- Sweep, then mop the floor with warm soapy water.

Bathroom

- Wash your shower curtain (check the cleaning label for which cycle to use.)
- Clean the soap scum and water spots from the shower doors and mirrors.
- Sort through the bathroom cabinets and clean the shelves.

- Use the toothbrush to scrub between the tiles, along the shower door tracks, and around the edge of the bath where mold and dirt build up.
- Mop the floor.

Living Room

- Remove and wash cushion covers and throw pillows, and vacuum the sofa and chairs thoroughly with the brush attachment for the vacuum cleaner. You can also run a lint roller over everything.
- Dust any photo frames and wipe the glass.
- Dust underneath any electronics.
- Dust the lampshades.
- Vacuum the curtains or blinds and wipe the windows and windowsills.
- Wipe the baseboards.
- Beat any rugs outside to remove loose dirt and dust, then vacuum the carpet and rugs thoroughly.

These tasks do not need to be done every week or even every month, but be sure to do them a few times a year, particularly in summer, when pollen, dust, and insects are everywhere. If you deep clean one room a month, you'll do them all three times a year!

Cleaning is one of the most important parts of your routine, not only for your health but also for your happiness. Routines, in general, give us structure and control, and in the next chapter, we'll look more closely at the ways routines impact and improve our lives and health.

9

A NEAT 7-DAY PACKAGE

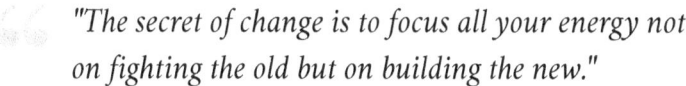

"The secret of change is to focus all your energy not on fighting the old but on building the new."

— SOCRATES, PHILOSOPHER

A s we have ventured our way through to the end of this book, we have stressed the importance of maintaining the strength and structure of your two pillars of power and stressed how vital they are to balance your life and happiness.

The pillars of your physical and mental health are indispensable to your power. Together they are the foundation of your entire being, and your life will be a difficult struggle without one or the other. The strength of both pillars is forged from the three main ingredients we covered in the preceding chapters. **Exercise**. **Nutrition**.

Sleep. Each piece plays such a vital role in building the strength of the pillars that they will begin to crack and crumble if one of them is unaccounted for.

Without proper exercise, your physical health diminishes, which can lead to anxiety and depression, therefore, affecting your mental health negatively. In turn, this can lead to poor eating habits and sleeping disorders.

Without proper nutrition, the body will not have the essential nutrients it needs to provide the energy required to exercise successfully and maintain a high level of physical health. Both pillars begin to crumble, and sleep is impacted yet once again.

Without proper sleep, you can abandon the thought of having optimal physical health and nutrition results. When you lack adequate sleep, you lack energy and are always tired and sluggish.

When you lack energy, you resist pushing harder toward committing to that exercise routine. You lack the energy to meal prep ahead of time, which ensures you are consuming a healthy and balanced diet. You resort to quick and ready meals and lounging on the couch. Countless hours of unproductive, wasted time is lost when you do not invest those crucial hours in sleeping. We both have been guilty of sacrificing sleep hours to gain productive work hours, and the trade-off is a heavier price to pay than we imagined.

The time to reign in your physical and mental health to supercharge your life is now, and we will show you how by invigorating your daily routines!

Routines rule our daily lives from the moment we wake up and stretch to the moment we hit the pillow yawning. So many of our behaviors and actions happen without thought because we are so accustomed to the routines we overlook. Sometimes this is great, like when your feet walk themselves home after a long shift so your mind can wander peacefully, but at other times routine can take over your life and prevent you from making necessary changes to your lifestyle or trying something new. They make us feel comfortable, but they can also trap us if they aren't occasionally refreshed or revamped to make room for new healthy routines. It's time to focus on building routines that will help you change your life and put you on the path to a healthier body and mind to being the best version of yourself.

ROUTINES

Routines are actions done at certain times or in a particular order, usually repeated daily or weekly. Your whole day is constructed around a series of routines within your routine. We have routines for everything, including morning routines, commuting to work or school, cleaning and cooking, shopping, showering, and going to bed. There are many benefits to keeping up with routines.

They can help us to stay organized and productive and assist us in completing tasks we would otherwise forget or procrastinate. They encourage you to achieve tasks and goals by setting aside time for them. Routines give structure to your day, so you can plan how to use your precious free time rather than wasting it, and having a system helps to create a calm environment because you know what to expect from your day.

When it comes to health, routines are instrumental in keeping up healthy habits and reaching your fitness goals:

- Routines help with stress management, reducing anxiety and heart disease risk.
- Morning and bedtime routines help to regulate your sleep cycle, improving your sleep hygiene and health and enabling you to wake up energized, with your body and mind rested and ready for the day.
- You can build healthy habits into your routine, like planning your trips to the grocery store rather than popping to the store when you're hungry, and planning time for healthy snacks into your routine will stop you from grazing or craving unhealthy snacks.
- Daily routines that make time for exercise will make a tremendous difference in your weight loss or fitness journey! Budgeting your time to allow for exercise means you are less likely to skip a

workout and won't feel like you have to rush through it.

- Incorporating meal planning into your routine will help you to eat a healthier diet because you can prepare for the day's meals in advance, rather than needing a quick-fix dinner—which often ends up being less than healthy—at the last moment.

Level Up Your Daily Routine

You can change up your daily routine at any time to make your day more productive or energizing—even small changes can make a huge difference as long as you commit. Here are some quick ideas to add to your daily routine to bring you a step closer to a healthy, happy, and balanced life.

Get Energized

Power up your day and get out of a slump with these routine rechargers:

- Drink a glass of room temperature water with a fresh lemon slice when you wake up—it will help improve digestion and refresh your body by removing toxins; while also giving you a boost of vitamin C.
- Work out in the morning to get your blood flowing and your muscles full of energy.

- Eat a nutritious breakfast every day.
- Stay hydrated by ensuring to drink plenty of water throughout your day.
- Eat an energizing lunch—avoid fatty foods, which can cause lethargy, and have a good dose of slow-release carbohydrates to get you through the afternoon.
- Stretch out the mid-afternoon slump! Our energy levels tend to drop around 3-4 p.m., so set up reminders to get up and stretch or take a quick walk when you feel the slump coming.
- Ditch the caffeine after 5 p.m.
- Have your dinner planned in advance so you can quickly throw together a healthy evening meal.
- Have another lemon water before going to bed at a reasonable hour.

Get Organized

Use these tips to bring a little more order and control to your busy life:

- Make your bed when you get up so you're less likely to crawl back into it and start your day in an organized mindset.
- Prepare your exercise outfits, work clothes, and work or gym bag the night before and lay them out ready for the morning.

- Wipe up behind yourself. After your shower, give the bathroom surfaces a quick wipe, and during and after cooking, do the same in the kitchen. Little and often cleaning is much easier than a big weekly clean that takes up half the weekend.
- Put things back where they belong when you're finished with them.
- Keep a grocery list on your fridge and add to it when you notice something is low so that you don't miss anything.
- Run an essential items check before you leave the house. Have you got your phone, keys, wallet, charger, employee ID, water bottle, etc.? Do this check every time you head out, and it will soon become a great habit.
- Prioritize your most important and urgent tasks for the day or week, and work your way through them first.
- Check your finances every morning and track your budget throughout the day.
- Do the dishes straight after dinner!

Be Productive

You can have a productive day every day if you shape your routine to work to your benefit!

- Plan your day the night before.
- Keep to the same bedtime and wake-up time every day.
- Declutter your workspace at the end of every day so that the next morning it is clear of distractions.
- Focus on your goals and priorities in the morning when your brain is most active and creative. Save emails and mind-numbing work for the afternoon.
- Tackle the most complex or the most urgent task first!
- Make time to *rest*—you could schedule a meditation or reading time in the afternoon to avoid burnout.
- Split your working day into 45-minute work sessions with 15-minute breaks between. Switch to another task for a while when you feel unproductive with a particular task.

Taking on all these habits may be overwhelming, so try slowly integrating them into your daily routine, one or a few at a time. One of the main reasons people struggle to keep to a routine is they make it too difficult or too packed with things to remember that they slip back into the easy old habits that weren't working for them either. Your routine shouldn't be so strict or cumbersome that when you miss a step, you feel like you have failed, as this can set up a negative mindset about your routine, making it more likely you won't keep to it. The key is to find balance in your routines to allow flexibility, set easy-to-follow patterns, and keep your routines realistically achievable.

Sticking to a Routine

Sticking to a new routine can be very challenging at first. You have to learn new behaviors and exercise your self-control more than you have been, which can make your new routine seem like more effort than it is worth. With time and perseverance, you'll find your routine easier and more rewarding, but how can you stick to it in those first few difficult weeks when it seems like your routine rules your every waking moment?

Firstly, it is fundamental to **remember *why* you changed your routine**. Keeping your initial motivations and goals in mind will keep you focused on the rewards for sticking to your routine and make the effort feel worthwhile. If you aim to create a productive weekday routine in order to be able to enjoy your weekends more, then keep that in mind when your to-do list seems daunting.

Next, **identify where you could improve the routine**. What area seems most arduous to maintain or integrate?

What part of your new routine keeps tripping you up? It may be that you find your unfamiliar early wake-up call a struggle or that you don't have time to cook the dinners you planned when you get home from work—find the weak spot and figure out a way to make it work rather than just giving up.

All the steps of your routine have a butterfly effect on each other, so if you start your day by waking up later than usual, it pushes back your whole day and can leave you rushing to finish tasks and playing catch-up. This in itself leads to added stress and demotivation, so the best way to stick to your routine is to **start the day on the front foot**. A good start makes a good day more likely!

Set a goal for sticking to your new routine. Set your plan that you'll keep laboring at it for two weeks. Check off the days you achieve it and track your progress to the end. If you miss a day, start over and see if you can do it for a solid two weeks the next time.

You can **keep a journal of how your new routine is working for you**. At the end of your busy day, wind down before bed by jotting down how your routine made you feel that day. What was strenuous, what really worked, and what are you hoping for the next day? Remind yourself of what your routine is working towards, and explore your feelings about your progress. You could also write down some **positive affirmations about your routine**, for example, "My routine makes me feel excited for the day!" or "Today was a very productive and successful day, and tomorrow will be too!"

There are many ways to make your routine work flawlessly every day. Ultimately, it all comes down to your willpower, self-control, and desire to stick to it and enjoy the benefits. Set the wheels in motion to force your routine to work for you and strive toward achieving your goals because they are crucial to taking control of your life.

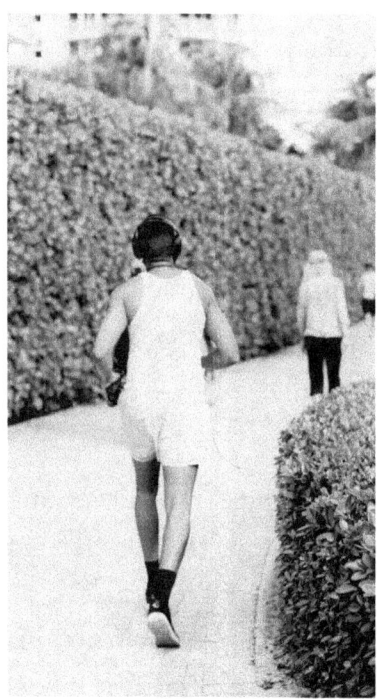

BUILDING THE BEST ROUTINE FOR THE BEST YOU

In a beautiful and uplifting article about struggling to stick to routines, Catherine Andrews wrote that "routines are an investment in yourself, and an act of self-love." (Andrews, 2018) When routines are viewed in this way, it is hard to find a reason *not* to invest in upgrading your routine to achieve your goals and improve your life. You deserve to enjoy the rewards and peace of mind of a healthy daily routine. After all, you work hard, and life is demanding enough without feeling unmotivated, distracted, and unproductive all the time. Seeing your routine as an act of self-love will help you to stick to it, knowing that you are gifting yourself time, energy, less stress, and better mental and physical health. You should be your own priority, and building a routine that prioritizes your health, goals, and values will improve your sense of self-worth and keep negative energy and influences out of your life.

Your routines should align your goals and direction across all areas, making time for fitness, reflection, self-care, and sleep. Think of each day of the week as a stepping stone to a better life. Every day should help you progress towards your goals, even if only in a tiny way, like sticking to your sleep schedule or taking the time to make a meal rather than ordering takeout. So, to build your new routines and daily schedule, keep your fitness, nutrition, and sleep goals in mind to ensure that you work towards them every day.

Let's build a goal-oriented routine for a 7-day stretch that could change your life in just a week! For each day, we'll add sleep, fitness, and nutrition elements—plus other areas—to gradually work up to a supercharged schedule one day at a time.

Sunday Night Checklist*

*For the week ahead, you'll need to get a notebook. Use half of the notebook to write your bedtime checklist, daily tasks, exercise plan, and meal plan, and the other half to keep a journal of reflections and notes on how the new routine works for you.

Start preparing for your new routine on a Sunday night, ready for the working week. Work through this checklist to get yourself in the perfect mindset for the changes and improvements to come!

1. After dinner, do the dishes straight away. Set a timer for 30 minutes and spend the time cleaning up the house, putting away laundry, and wiping down the kitchen and bathroom surfaces. Open your bedroom window and change your bed sheets.
2. Pour yourself a soothing cup of tea, take out paper and a pen, and make a list of the things

you need to do tomorrow. Then, put those things in order of importance so your tasks are prioritized—you'll be doing this exercise every night for the next week.

3. Next, plan your meals—breakfast, lunch, and dinner—for the whole next week, and make a grocery list. Include a few healthy snacks on the list. Go through your cabinets, fridge, and freezer to see what you already have in the house, and make use of that first!

4. Now plan an exercise session for 30 minutes each day, for example:

    a. Monday: Morning yoga (20 minutes), lunchtime walk (10 minutes)

    b. Tuesday: Morning Pilates (30 minutes)

    c. Wednesday: Morning jog (20 minutes), lunchtime yoga (10 minutes)

Give yourself two days when you take a gentle walk instead of a workout. You don't want to avoid exercise altogether, but "rest" days of low-intensity exercise will keep your body stronger than if you do nothing at all.

5. Prepare your exercise and work clothes for the morning and pack your work bag. Put a glass of water by your bed.

6. Around 9.30 p.m., start your sleep hygiene routine.

This Sunday night routine will kickstart the whole week to come and sets up some good habits from the beginning!

7-Day Supercharge

Use this routine as a template for every day this week— you can add and change things for each day, such as your exercises and meals, but it should keep to a similar order to help you build up good habits.

Morning:

- 7 a.m.: Wake up and have a quick stretch in bed. Don't lie around scrolling through social media— get straight up!
- Drink some water with fresh lemon.
- Do 20-30 minutes of exercise.
- Have a quick shower and dress for work.
- Eat a nutritious breakfast, e.g., oatmeal, scrambled eggs, or fruit and yogurt.
- Prepare a healthy lunch to take to work, ideally something with protein to aid concentration.
- Now you can check your phone and go to work!

Afternoon:

- At lunchtime, try to get in 10-15 minutes of gentle exercise—go for a walk, do some quick cardio exercises, or stretch at your desk.
- Eat your lunch and drink water.
- **Monday:** On your way home from work, do a food shop for everything you'll need for the week's meals.

Evening:

- Prepare and eat your dinner.
- Do the dishes and wipe down the kitchen.
- Spend an hour working towards one of your career, personal growth, or spiritual goals, or if you didn't have time for morning exercise, now is the time to do it!
- Now you can unwind with some TV or a hobby.
- Have a quick clean up and open the bedroom window.
- Write down your tasks for tomorrow, and set out your work clothes and bag.
- In your journal, write about how your new routine feels each day. Was it fun? How did it make you feel? How did your day improve? What changes felt easiest or most meddlesome? Take some time to reflect.

Bedtime:

- Start your sleep hygiene routine around 9.30 p.m.

  - Dim all the lights, and put on some soothing music.
  - Take a warm bath or shower.
  - Do your skincare routine and get into your pajamas.
  - Set your alarm for 7 a.m. and then turn off your phone wifi, lower your phone screen brightness, and put your phone on the other side of the room across from your bed.
  - Get into bed with a book and read for at least half an hour—if you choose a book that aligns with one of your goals, even better!
  - Drink some water.
  - Turn off your light by 11 p.m.

The purpose of this routine is to incorporate all the elements of this book into your week, enabling you to meet your goals, break bad habits, and improve your mental and physical health. It makes time for every facet of the two pillars and fills your day with healthy habits promoting self-care, progress, and wellness. After a week of this routine, you should feel energized and productive and like you've started on the right path for the life and future you hope for. Sticking to this routine in the long term and, in time, expanding and improving it will be an incredibly considerable learning experience.

Now you're ready to start your new routine, all that remains is to commit to taking back control of your life and focusing your energy on strengthening the two essential pillars of existence so that they can support you in all your endeavors, adventures, hopes, and dreams.

BEFORE YOU PUT YOUR SNEAKERS ON...

If this book has helped you understand the connection between your physical and mental health, and inspired you to prioritize both in your daily life, we hope you can do us a favor and leave a quick review on Amazon.

Share your thoughts on the 7-day supercharge and let them know how it made you feel. We would love to hear how this easy-to-follow routine impacted everything from your mood to your sleep.

WANT TO HELP OTHERS?

Thank you for your support. We are so looking forward to someone reading your words and deciding that this is the day they will take their health into their hands and put an end to bad habits standing in the way of success.

Scan the QR code for a quick review!

CONCLUSION

Working to improve your mental and physical health, to strengthen and build upon your two pillars, is a lifetime commitment that will bring purpose, clarity, and confidence into your life. The two pillars are the source of your energy and potential. Throughout life, you will draw on them every single day to achieve your goals, enjoy your endeavors, and face your challenges—this is why keeping them and yourself strong, stable, and supported is the most important thing you can do.

Your mental health is your compass, your internal guide that tells you what you want and need, who you are, and who you could be, and with care and attention, it can be an endless source of strength and energy. There is no limit to what you can achieve if you take care of your mind and encourage happiness and mental stability in your life. Your physical health and your body are your toolkits for life, your vessel through thick and thin, and this vessel, like any other, must be cared for, kept clean, healthy, and strong to make journeys and face the world's weather. With self-love and care, your body will carry you through life and open up a world of energy and adventure. It will walk you along the beach, climb mountains, carry your children, and so much more, bringing you to the places and experiences that will fill your life with joy and excitement. Pay attention to how your body feels and give it what it *needs*, not what it *wants*, and keep working towards a fitter, stronger, healthier body and a more fulfilling and enjoyable life.

There may be days in the future when, no matter how excellent your routines or habits are or how well you've slept or eaten, you feel unmotivated, demoralized, or unproductive and have wasted all your effort and sunk back into your old patterns and habits. It happens to everyone, and it doesn't mean you have failed or wasted your efforts—one crummy day mustn't deprive you of a hundred good days! Believe in yourself! You know who you are and no one else can take that away from you.

Come back to this book and remind yourself that you *can* do it. You *can* keep moving forward with simple changes and a positive mindset. Go back to your to-do list and pick one thing to get done, or drop something that's overwhelming you and do a meditation or some self-care to help you reset and regroup within yourself. Be honest about what is working and not working for you, and keep finding ways to change and improve that draw you closer to your goals. The trials and temptations of our modern world are a constant challenge to our mental and physical health, but to rise to that challenge and overcome it will strengthen your two pillars and give you a firm base for building a rewarding and happy life.

The book may be over, but your journey is just beginning. It is never too late to take the reins of your life and get on track to a better life and a better you. Taking back control of your life by breaking bad habits, supercharging your routine, and improving your mental and physical health takes courage, determination, and strength of will. By simply seeking a path to a better life, you have decided to put yourself first and gift yourself the life you deserve. You deserve to enjoy the rewards for your efforts, achieve your goals and dreams, and build an extraordinary life of adventure and joy. So, what are you waiting for? Get out there and use your new knowledge and skills to reinvigorate your life!

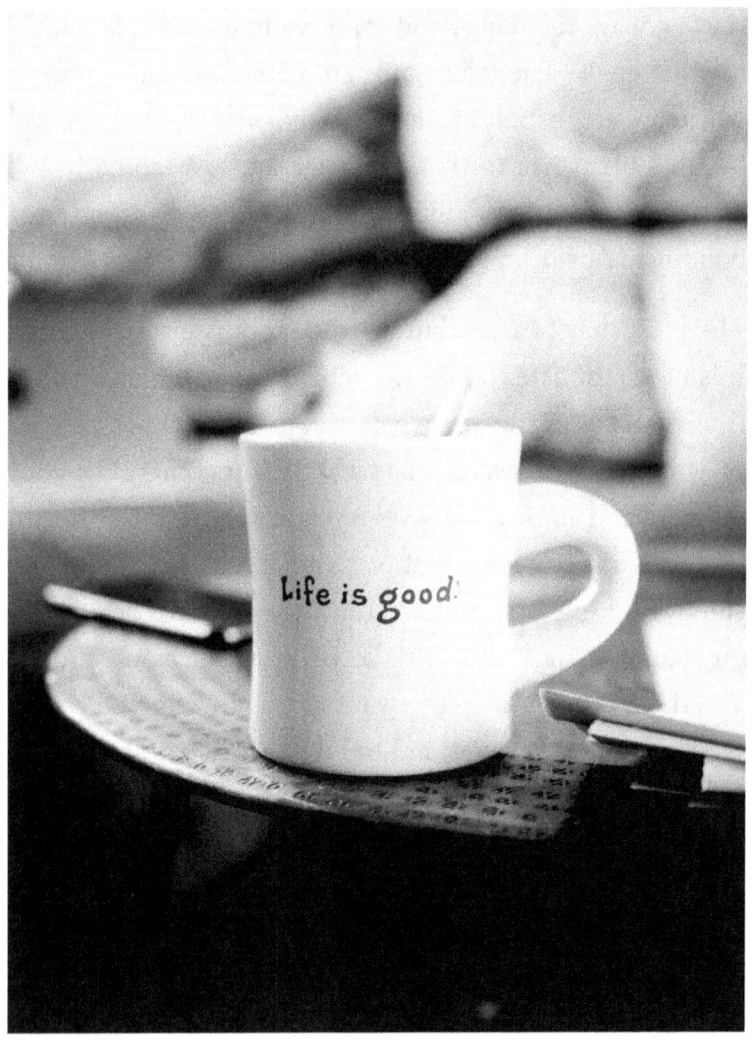

JUST FOR YOU!

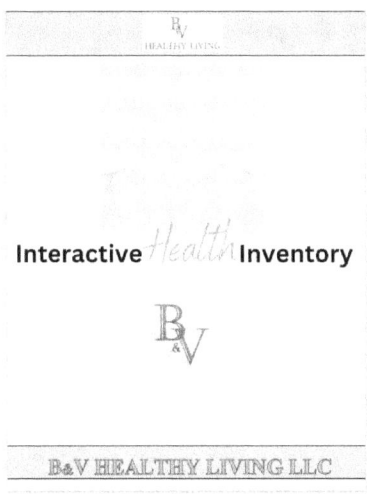

Interactive Health Inventory

B&V HEALTHY LIVING LLC

A FREE GIFT TO OUR READERS
Download and print the **Two Pillars of Power:
Interactive Health Inventory**

The Health Inventory should be used as you progress
through each chapter assessing your current health and
setting new goals that will transform your life right away!
Visit the link:

https://bvhealthyliving.org/HealthInventory

REFERENCES

Altrogge, S. (2022, December). *12 morning and evening routines that will set up each day for success.* Zapier. https://zapier.com/blog/daily-routines/

Andrews, C. (2018, May 7). *I used to struggle with routines until I figured this out.* Medium. https://candrews.medium.com/struggling-with-sticking-to-routines-it-might-be-for-a-different-reason-than-you-think-e0378828182

Aronov-Jacoby, S. (2022, January 27). *The benefits of self-awareness.* Humber River Hospital. https://www.hrh.ca/2022/01/27/the-bene fits-of-self-awareness/

Bennett, J. (2022, December 20). *This room-by-room guide makes deep cleaning your house so much easier.* Better Homes & Gardens. https://www.bhg.com/homekeeping/house-cleaning/tips/how-to-deep-clean-your-house/

Betz, M. (2022, September 14). *What is self-awareness, and why is it important?* BetterUp. https://www.betterup.com/blog/what-is-self-awareness

Bhatt Patel, R. (2021, July 16). *6 unexpected ways decluttering can help you destress, calm down, and take care of your mental health.* Apartment Therapy. https://www.apartmenttherapy.com/mental-health-bene fits-decluttering-36948599

Bjarnadottir, A. (2021, November 2). *25 simple tips to make your diet healthier.* Healthline. https://www.healthline.com/nutrition/healthy-eating-tips#TOC_TITLE_HDR_10

Boksic, B. (2014, March 24). *What is a routine? 9 ways to define a routine that works.* Lifehack. https://www.lifehack.org/articles/productiv ity/why-using-routines-will-make-you-more-productive.html

Boulos, Dr. M. (2020, May 21). *Your healthy sleep checklist.* Heart and Stroke Foundation of Canada. https://www.heartandstroke.ca/arti cles/your-healthy-sleep-checklist

Brennan, D. (2021, March). *How does mental health affect physical health.*

WebMD. https://www.webmd.com/mental-health/how-does-mental-health-affect-physical-health

CDC. (2021, January 4). *How does sleep affect your heart health?* Centers for Disease Control and Prevention. https://www.cdc.gov/blood pressure/sleep.htm

CDC. (2022, September 13). *Sleep hygiene tips - sleep and sleep disorders.* Centers for Disease Control and Prevention; Centers for Disease Control and Prevention. https://www.cdc.gov/sleep/about_sleep/ sleep_hygiene.html

Centers for Disease Control and Prevention. (2022, June 16). *Benefits of physical activity.* Centers for Disease Control and Prevention; CDC. https://www.cdc.gov/physicalactivity/basics/pa-health/index. htm#:

Cherry, K. (2023, March 10). *What Is self-awareness?* Verywell Mind. https://www.verywellmind.com/what-is-self-awareness-2795023

Clear, J. (2013, May 13). *How to break a bad habit (and replace it with a good one).* James Clear. https://jamesclear.com/how-to-break-a-bad-habit

Covey, S. R. (2004). *The 7 habits of highly effective people: Powerful lessons in personal change.* Free Press.

Eatough, E. (2021, December 7). *How to form good habits (and ditch bad ones)* BetterUp. https://www.betterup.com/blog/building-habits

Eurich, T. (2018). *What self-awareness really is (and how to cultivate it).* Harvard Business Review; hbr.org. https://hbr.org/2018/01/what-self-awareness-really-is-and-how-to-cultivate-it

Felman, A. (2020, April 19). *Health: What does good health really mean?* Medical News Today. https://www.medicalnewstoday.com/arti cles/150999#types

Ferreira, M. (2018). *6 essential nutrients: What they are and why you need them.* Healthline. https://www.healthline.com/health/food-nutri tion/six-essential-nutrients

Gomstyn, A. (2019). *Food for your mood: How what you eat affects your mental health.* Aetna; Aetna. https://www.aetna.com/health-guide/ food-affects-mental-health.html

Gordon, S. (2021, February 23). *Mental health benefits of cleaning and decluttering*. Verywell Mind. https://www.verywellmind.com/how-mental-health-and-cleaning-are-connected-5097496

Headspace. (n.d.). *Sleep hygiene tips*. Headspace. Retrieved June 19, 2023, from https://www.headspace.com/sleep/sleep-hygiene

Ho, L. (2018, March 5). *Powerful daily routine examples for a healthy and high-achieving you*. Lifehack. https://www.lifehack.org/677367/powerful-daily-routine

Homemakers. (2020, October 1). *7 Benefits of a clean and organized home*. Homemakers.com. https://www.homemakers.com/blog/ideas-and-advice/7-benefits-of-a-clean-and-organized-home.html

Jones, R. (2023). 57 Self-Awareness quotes to Know Yourself Better. *Happier Human*. https://www.happierhuman.com/self-awareness-quotes/

Konga Fitness. (n.d.). Best exercise and mental health quotes to get you through the week. https://kongafitness.com/best-exercise-and-mental-health-quotes-to-get-you-through-the-week/

Keenan, M. (2022, December 1). *200+ Motivational Quotes To Inspire and Win 2023*. Shopify. https://www.shopify.com/blog/motivational-quotes

Kristenson, S. (2022, May 5). *7 benefits of setting & achieving SMART goals*. Develop Good Habits. https://www.developgoodhabits.com/benefits-smart-goals/

Lim, S. (2020, May 8). *7 things you should do when you fail to achieve your goals*. Stunning Motivation. https://stunningmotivation.com/fail-achieve-goals/

Marks, J. L. (2023, April 26). *How to clean your house if depression is getting in your way*. Everyday Health. https://www.everydayhealth.com/depression/clean-house-when-youre-depressed.aspx

Mayo Clinic. (2018). *Infectious diseases - Symptoms and causes*. Mayo Clinic. https://www.mayoclinic.org/diseases-conditions/infectious-diseases/symptoms-causes/syc-20351173

Mental Health Foundation. (2022, February 18). *Physical health and mental health*. Mentalhealth.org. https://www.mentalhealth.org.uk/explore-mental-health/a-z-topics/physical-health-and-mental-health#:

Milkman, K. (2021, November 29). *How to build a habit in 5 steps, according to science.* CNN. https://edition.cnn.com/2021/11/29/health/5-steps-habit-builder-wellness/index.html

Mind Tools. (2022). *SMART Goals.* Mind Tools. https://www.mindtools.com/a4wo118/smart-goals

Mueller, S. (2023, January 1). *How to (finally) break that bad habit.* Wired. https://www.wired.com/story/how-to-break-bad-habits/

National Eating Disorders Association. (2018a, February 22). *Warning signs and symptoms.* National Eating Disorders Association. https://www.nationaleatingdisorders.org/warning-signs-and-symptoms

National Institute of Mental Health. (2023, March). *Mental illness.* National Institute of Mental Health. https://www.nimh.nih.gov/health/statistics/mental-illness

News In Health. (2017, May 31). *The benefits of slumber* (H. Wein, Ed.). NIH News in Health. https://newsinhealth.nih.gov/2013/04/benefits-slumber#:

NHS. (2022, February 24). *8 tips for healthy eating.* NHS. https://www.nhs.uk/live-well/eat-well/how-to-eat-a-balanced-diet/eight-tips-for-healthy-eating/

NHSinform. (2022, August 26). *Chronic pain.* NHSinform. https://www.nhsinform.scot/illnesses-and-conditions/brain-nerves-and-spinal-cord/chronic-pain#:

Page, S. (2021, February 8). 27 Inspirational Health Quotes to Motivate Employees. *Employee Wellness Blog.* Retrieved July 23, 2023, from https://info.totalwellnesshealth.com/blog/27-inspirational-health-quotes

Parker-Pope, T. (2020, February 18). *How to build healthy habits.* The New York Times. https://www.nytimes.com/2020/02/18/well/mind/how-to-build-healthy-habits.html

Perkal, Z. (2015, August 31). *30 ways to brighten your daily routine.* Wanderlust. https://wanderlust.com/journal/30-ways-to-brighten-your-daily-routine/

Pietrangelo, A. (2019, January 15). *How to be happy: 25 habits to add to your routine.* Healthline; Healthline Media. https://www.healthline.com/health/how-to-be-happy#daily-habits

Polar. (2019, June 18). *9 ways to make time for exercise with a busy sched-*

ule. Polar. https://www.polar.com/blog/9-ways-how-to-make-time-for-exercise/

Ra0, J. (2023, Jul6). *25 Awesome Quotes On Nutrition*. STYLECRAZE. https://www.stylecraze.com/articles/awesome-quotes-on-nutrition/

Raypole, C. (2019, October 29). *How to break a habit: 15 tips for success*. Healthline. https://www.healthline.com/health/how-to-break-a-habit#prepare-for-slipups

Riopel, L. (2019, September 14). *17 self-awareness activities and exercises (+ test)*. Positive Psychology. https://positivepsychology.com/self-awareness-exercises-activities-test/#questions

Saber Healthcare. (2021, March 9). *7 ways to improve your diet & nutrition*. Saber Healthcare. https://www.saberhealth.com/news/blog/improve-your-nutrition

Scallon, T. (2020, June 26). *Essential nutrients*. St. Luke's Health. https://www.stlukeshealth.org/resources/essential-nutrients#:

Selhub, E. (2022, September 18). *Nutritional psychiatry: Your brain on food*. Harvard Health Blog; Harvard Health Publishing. https://www.health.harvard.edu/blog/nutritional-psychiatry-your-brain-on-food-201511168626

Semeco, A. (2017, February 10). *The top 10 benefits of regular exercise*. Healthline. https://www.healthline.com/nutrition/10-benefits-of-exercise#TOC_TITLE_HDR_11

Sherrell, Z. (2021, November 30). *5 neurological disorders: Symptoms explained*. Medical News Today. https://www.medicalnewstoday.com/articles/neurological-disorders

Sievers, M. (2020). 101 of the best sleep quotes + wall prints. *Casper Blog*. https://casper.com/blog/sleep-quotes/

Sleep Center of Middle Tennessee . (2019, April 4). *Get better sleep tonight with simple bedroom "spring cleaning."* Sleep Center of Middle Tennessee. https://sleepcenterinfo.com/blog/bedroom-spring-cleaning/#:

SokyaHealth. (2021, January 7). *Good nutrition for mental and physical health*. SokyaHealth. https://www.sokyahealth.com/thrive/the-importance-of-good-nutrition-for-mental-and-physical-health/

Stutter Health. (2019). *Eating well for mental health*. Sutterhealth.org.

https://www.sutterhealth.org/health/nutrition/eating-well-for-mental-health

Suni, E. (2020, August 14). *What is sleep hygiene?* (N. Vyas, Ed.). Sleep Foundation. https://www.sleepfoundation.org/sleep-hygiene

Suni, E. (2021, December 2). *Stages of sleep: What happens in a sleep cycle* (N. Vyas, Ed.). Sleep Foundation. https://www.sleepfoundation.org/stages-of-sleep

Suni, E., & Dimitriu, A. (2020, September 18). *Mental health and sleep.* Sleep Foundation; Sleep Foundation. https://www.sleepfoundation.org/mental-health

Thomas, A. (2022, April 19). *Dangers of diet culture.* Norman Regional Health System. https://www.normanregional.com/blog/dangers-of-diet-culture

Wild, M. (2018, June 8). *How to design your kitchen to eat Healthier - Debbie Rodrigues.* Debbie Rodrigues. https://debbieinshape.com/how-to-design-your-kitchen-to-eat-healthier/

Williams, T. (n.d.). *Bad habits: Definition, examples, and how to break them.* The Berkeley Well-Being Institute. Retrieved June 24, 2023, from https://www.berkeleywellbeing.com/bad-habits.html

World Health Organization. (2022, June 8). *Mental disorders.* World Health Organization. https://www.who.int/news-room/fact-sheets/detail/mental-disorders

Wix Answers *(2022, January 6). 50 inspiring quotes on business growth and Success. WIX Answers.* https://www.wixanswers.com/post/business-growth-quotes

Yuko, E. (2023, January 24). *12 home decor tips for a mental health boost.* Real Simple. https://www.realsimple.com/home-decor-for-mental-health-7098644#:

IMAGE REFERENCES

All images sourced on Unsplash.